AVOID THE
AGING
TRAP

66 In this century in which we have prolonged life so remarkably, we need Dr. Oberleder's new, wise and lucid book to help us deal with this special stage of life. 99

Robert N. Butler M.D.
Former Director
National Institute on Aging
National Institutes of Health

AVOID THE
AGING
TRAP

Muriel Oberleder, Ph.D.
Internationally known gerontologist
and clinical psychologist

ACROPOLIS BOOKS LTD.
Washington, D.C.

ACROPOLIS BOOKS LTD.
Colortone Building, 2400 17th St., N.W.,
Washington, D.C. 20009

Printed in the United States of America by
COLORTONE PRESS Creative Graphics, Inc.
Washington, D.C. 20009

Library of Congress Cataloging in Publication Data

Oberleder, Muriel.
  Avoid the aging trap.
  Includes index.
  1. Aging—Psychological aspects. 2. Old
age. 3. Aged—Psychology. I Title.
HQ1061.023 1982   305.2'6   82-11472
ISBN 0-87491-496-5

For My Significant Others

Contents

Chapter One
You Can Teach
An Old Dog New Tricks

7

Chapter Two
The Myth of Senility

Chapter Three
Memory Loss May Be
Good for You

Chapter Four
Problem Parents of Middle-Aged Children And Vice Versa

69

Chapter Five
Those Golden Anniversary Blues!

85

Chapter Six
Dealing With Depression in Everyday Life

Chapter Seven
Food, Friends, Exercise— The Big Three of Aging

Chapter Eight
Swinging After Sixty   145

Chapter Nine
What Kind Of Old Person
Will You Be?   163

Chapter Ten
Meet the New Elderly 179

Selected Bibliography 199

Index 208

Introduction

*"If I had known that I would live this long,
I would have taken better care of myself."*
—Anon.

Humans have been programmed to stay alive for at least one hundred years—and these days more and more of us are making it!

People are living longer and feeling younger than ever before. With the percentage of the population over sixty-five increasing each year, it is time we took a long, hard look at the myths of aging which still predict "senility" after sixty—and, if we live long enough, eventually being "put away" in some nursing home.

All that you will be reading in this book has one goal: to explode the myths about aging. All the material in this book is based on current studies, surveys, and reports of people over sixty as they are today and as they are projected to be in the future.

You will recognize many of the ideas as simple, basic truths—that are true of yourself and of older people you have known. Other ideas will surprise you. You may even find it hard to believe them because, they seem *too* good to be true!

We have all been brainwashed into believing the myths.

"Finished" at Forty?

Even Sigmund Freud believed that psychoanalysis would be wasted on people over forty: he said they were too old to change, and anyway, the treatment took too long to make it worthwhile.

Today, people in their seventies and even eighties undergo analysis successfully, and in a fraction of the time it usually takes younger people! (Freud himself worked until his death in his eighties.)

Until the 1950's, the term "aging" rarely appeared in textbook indexes. Problems that occurred over the age of sixty were labeled "senility" or "chronic brain syndrome," and "arteriosclerosis" was the catchall diagnosis for a myriad of symptoms.

Aging was considered a disease. That this "disease" might be manmade, and reversible as well as preventable, was rarely considered. Today it is common knowledge.

"Senility"—A Psychosomatic Disease

Early in the century, the great psychiatrist, Carl Jung was deeply interested in the aging process. He was among the first to suspect that the stresses of life rather than the years themselves cause many of the problems of aging.

Jung regarded "senility" as a psychosomatic disease and the body's most overworked organ, the brain as highly susceptible to breakdown under stress. He also believed the brain is *capable of recovery when stress is removed.*

Why wasn't Jung heeded? Why did people cling to the idea that aging meant inevitable, irreversible losses? Was it possible that the diagnosis of "senility" was needed—as a garbage pail in which to dump the problems of aging?

Sandor Ferenczi, a contemporary of Freud and Jung, believed that this was so, and that it conveniently discouraged the search for other causes that *could* be treated. Today, although the situation is improving dramatically, many professions, and even the government, are still unconsciously negative about aging. Or perhaps even consciously negative, since nobody likes to be reminded of growing old—even the aging themselves.

Mind and Body Are One

When I began to work with the aging some thirty years ago as a clinical psychologist, I soon learned that the effects of body on mind and of mind on body are often indistinguishable. Frustration can cause poor health, as well as the loss of memory. And poor health can cause both.

I realized that it was necessary to view the *total* person against the background of his entire life, his place in society, and his society's place in time.

Like my colleagues I was trained in the myths of aging, which I have been unlearning ever since. I like to think that I was among those who helped to break the stranglehold of stereotypes and misconceptions about aging that have contaminated our attitudes. What a struggle it was.

But what rewards! Today, older people are involved in assertiveness training, consciousness-raising, and sex therapy rather than settling for "senility." As I learn from my older patients, I marvel at their resilience and recovery powers.

But many studies of aging still go the old route,

looking for weaknesses rather than strengths, for sickness rather than health. No wonder the results of these studies often contradict the observable realities of aging.

Test-Tube Aging

Aging is not a simple process to be studied in a laboratory experiment; it is a total, dynamic process that changes from person to person, place to place, and even within the same person from one situation to another. People grow old—and young again.

Yet, the bulk of our knowledge about the aging process comes from studies of old people in hospitals and nursing homes, or from comparisons of the aging with college students. Researchers seem to develop tunnel vision when they deal with the aging. Can it be that there is a vested interest in perpetuating the myths of aging?

The test-tube approach to aging means a special focus on symptoms or specific behaviors. But what about the feelings that cause the symptoms and behaviors in the first place?

Freud proved that the repression of anger, fear, and sexuality can cause havoc with mind, body, and behavior, and we will discuss this at length in relation to many so-called "problems" of aging.

The great danger of "test-tube aging" is that it promotes repression: it is easier to focus on the fact, say, that eighty-year-olds do not memorize nonsense syllables as well as twenty-year-olds than to face one's own dread of old age. And it is just this kind of repression that unconsciously affects us from the time we are young—making us unprepared for the time we are old.

The Aging Trap

How will you avoid the aging trap? By facing the facts and planning ahead.

Oddly enough, it is more difficult to face the good facts than the bad. When we are younger, and especially when we are middle-aged, we cannot believe that anything *good* can be associated with aging. We concentrate on the worst—that is if we let ourselves think about it at all.

As a student, I remember reading a report that a considerable percentage of people over sixty stated they were experiencing the most satisfying years of their lives. I thought they had to be kidding or were being Pollyannas.

Don't fall into that trap either. Many older people *are* enjoying their lives, although sometimes they may not admit it. And we will go into the reasons for that, too.

Middle-age is the prime time to plan for a happy old age. It is to old age as childhood is to adolescence, and adolescence is to adulthood. It should be a time of looking ahead and preparing—preparing an environment and a way of life that will provide opportunities for satisfying activities—ones that are conducive to self-respect.

What Kind of Old Person Will You Be?

Open, spontaneous, accepting of others, self-accepting, and above all, free of those hang-ups that held you back when you were younger. . .

Impossible, you say? Not only is it possible, but it is easier than you think. I hope that reading this book will convince you.

At the very least, you will not accept those myths about aging again. You may learn to cherish, enjoy, and express certain thoughts and feelings you thought were inappropriate for your age. You may exercise the talents you always had—and still have—in managing your life, even to the point of telling off those who "know what's best for you."

Most important, your real personality will be allowed to emerge when you develop new attitudes toward aging. And younger people may begin to see that older age is not so bad after all.

Chapter One

You Can Teach an Old Dog New Tricks

"...he grows old daily learning something new."

Cicero

Whoever coined the saying "You cannot teach an old dog new tricks" never owned a dog—and did not know very much about old people.

The myth that old people cannot learn new things is just that—myth. Today, older people are learning astrophysics, digital electronics, and modern business methods. And that is only with the left hemisphere of the brain! With the right hemisphere they are learning aerobic conditioning, Chinese brush-painting, and meditation.

Age is no barrier to learning, and universities around the world are opening their doors to older people. In fact, many colleges depend on the older student to keep not only enrollment up but their academic standards as well!

Of course, we all know the stereotype—somebody's uncle or aunt, past seventy, slowly slipping into dotage.

19

But old people *can* remain alert, physically active, valuable citizens. We can point to just a few examples—Grandma Moses, Bernard Baruch, Jack LaLanne, Gloria Swanson, George Burns.

These are exceptions, you say: after fifty we are on steep downgrade mentally.

Don't believe it! Let's take a look at the facts, not the myths. There is learning after sixty-five, lots of it.

Stimulation and Closure: Key to Learning

Exactly how and why we learn is a mystery, but it is certain that we cannot learn without stimulation. And once stimulated, we cannot relax until we have learned. When people are interrupted at a learning task, studies show, they will go back to it again and again. If they are not allowed to complete it, anxiety and irritability will mount, interfering with other future learning.

We need a feeling of completion, or "closure," in order to learn. The reward of satisfaction when a task is completed is what motivates and stimulates us. People who are constantly frustrated in their drive for closure begin to *avoid* stimulation, experiencing it as a dangerous feeling.

The reason many old people seem to voluntarily withdraw from the mainstream of life, as noted gerontologist Bernice Neugarten pointed out, is that isolation *protects* them from the "danger" of stimulation.

Of course, the old person pays a high price for this kind of "protection." We all know what isolation does to both young and old, and it is probably what happened to that dotty uncle and aunt.

Until a generation or two ago, the static lives of most old people were reflected in a learning deficiency that really has nothing to do with old age. But this provided a basis for the myth—the myth that has such a hold, even though the modern generation of older people is disproving it every day.

Why Older People Malfunction

The psychological study of older people is rather new, although this is not to say that the elderly have been ignored historically. Many excellent observations have been made since Cicero wrote his famous essays on aging.

But in the world of science, paradoxically, the stereotypes of aging have been paramount influences. Of course, there is a good reason for this: science studies things as they are; and older people very often fit the stereotypes, at least on the surface.

Successful adaptation to old age requires that "well-adjusted" people behave in ways they are expected to. Society *expects* older people to be less creative, less flexible, less capable of learning. "Normal" older people who are responsive to their society's tenets also expect it, since "good adjustment" means the ability to live within the limitations old age is supposed to impose on the individual.

Thus, a misconception created by society becomes a reality and reinforces the stereotype, which is why most scientific studies focus on what older people *cannot* do rather than on what they *can* do.

Most skills hold up very well with age; and many of those that don't can be made to. Society pays a heavy price for the unused talents of its older citizens.

The Lab-to-Life Controversy

The tests many employers give to younger workers simply do not apply to older workers, who may be highly qualifed for the job even though they cannot pass the test. These may be tests of memory—memorizing nonsense syllables, that is—or tapping levers at a given signal. In other words, the tests are usually "meaningless" in a practical sense; and while they may not faze a twenty-year-old, they may confuse and embarrass a person of sixty.

However, if older people are given time to orient themselves and practice a bit, they usually catch up in the areas that count. They may never match the young person in remembering nonsense syllables like "arg," "glup," and "clag" in the proper order, but there will be far fewer errors in their actual work, and their attendance records will beat the younger person's every time.

Such tests are so geared towards the negative as far as older people are concerned that the researchers (usually very young) often miss a good person even when they see one.

An important fact that emerges in almost all tests of memory is that *recognition memory* does not deteriorate with age. Old people may have trouble with names and recalling facts out of context but they always recognize them when they see them again.

This means that older people do learn new things that they store permanently in the brain, but that a clue or a reminder may be necessary to bring the information out. That is true at least on a *lab* test. In real life situations, they may not need reminding at all. If they haven't done something for a while they may need time to bone up, to practice. But who doesn't?

Lab studies do show that the older person benefits much more from practice than a young person. And if embarrassment and anxiety can be overcome before starting the test, the older person may not even have to practice at all.

Emotional Reactions to Learning Tests

Even the most carefully controlled test cannot control the emotional reactions an older person has, simply due to being put to the test—and by a younger person to boot.

Almost all weaknesses that show up—slower response, initial difficulty when questions are first presented, the problem of immediate recall—can be attributed to emotional reactions.

In a sense, the older person is being put on the spot by a younger person, who is making a comparison between younger and older people. Considering older people's own self-doubts (don't forget, they also share the stereotypes), it's remarkable that they can function at all.

Two things happen. First, the test situation becomes a stress situation, and we know what anxiety does to someone who is already on the spot. Second, the older person becomes angry and resentful, and of course, represses these feelings—which affects learning.

In an experiment on learning, one group of students was deliberately angered by an argumentative instructor who used high-handed, arbitrary methods. A second group of students was exposed to a kind, friendly instructor. You guessed it. Those students who were angered did very poorly, particularly in memory, attention, and problem-solving. Later, when they were being "debriefed," they described how their anger prevented them from "thinking straight." The other group had no problems in learning.

What's Your Anxiety Level?

Anxiety comes in many forms. Some are easily recognized—other signs are more subtle. Here is a list of cues which tell us that we are anxious. Check off those that you have experienced. When they occur again, you'll know that it's time to step back, calm down, and start over.

- Irritability
- Shoulder tense
- Got to go to bathroom
- Chest feels heavy
- Mouth dry
- Can't concentrate
- Anger
- Neck tense
- Voice sounds trembly
- Hard to draw a deep breath
- Hands cold

- Voice higher
- Heart beats fast
- Feel like crying

- Talk faster
- Confused
- Can't stop fidgeting

Effects of Stress

While young people are affected by test anxiety, the older person is more vulnerable to stress, and more likely to "regress" in performance; that is, to go back to behavior learned earlier in life. Regression is a natural defense under stress.

Think of yourself in stressful situations. How often have you forgotten the mature things you know and acted childishly instead? Under stress, all of us turn back to earlier, not later learned behavior.

This applies to reasoning as well. You may be perfectly capable of high-level reasoning, but in a stress condition you may reason at a lower level, sometimes foolishly. This only means you are under stress; it doesn't mean you have become a fool.

One test of reasoning starts with a simple question such as, "How are an apple and an orange alike?" A child might answer, "They are both round." An adult should answer, "They are both fruit." An older person may not answer at all, or argue that they are not alike, and may respond similarly to all the simple questions (thus earning the poor scores that fuel the learning myth). But after the test is over, that person will answer all the difficult questions correctly.

What has happened to cause the return of reason? First, there has been time to overcome anxiety and understand what is expected. Second, each simple question had a practice effect. Finally, the older person puts it all together and comes up with the right answers to the really difficult questions. You may be sure, the next time that test or one like it is given, this person will sail right through.

There are other differences between young and old that have nothing to do with capacity. When a test is timed, the older person may "freeze," fearing failure more than he or she is seeking success. This means the older person may become overcautious and refuse to take risks. If you're afraid to take a guess, you have less chances of being right.

Sometimes fear will lead a person to give "crazy" answers, because we may see things the way we need to see them. All of us tend to alter reality to fit our needs, but it may happen more often to older people, especially on tests, because their egos are more "at risk."

Why Old and Young Need Feedback

The principle is the same for people of all ages. Anyone who is put on the spot may become irrational in arguments. This is usually corrected by feedback: someone gives you another point of view, and subsequent experience brings you back to normal reasoning.

But feedback is often denied to the elderly, because people don't want to bother giving them another point of view, or they may not want to upset them and so will give false feedback. "Ah, well, I'll just play along." Or they may simply be respectful: after all, we are taught not to contradict our elders. But this hardly helps an older person to get back on the track!

Of course feedback is a two-way business. Nobody relishes being wrong, and many older people, because they are so vulnerable, resent it. In fact, some may choose to bow out altogether (this is called disengagement), rather than remain involved—and subject to criticism.

The problem is, without normal give-and-take a person lives in a vacuum. That is why an old person seems to lose the ability to learn. On laboratory test which provide feedback as the test proceeds ("the answer to 'A' was wrong, try 'B' or 'C'"), the differences in learning ability between young and old disappear.

Reactivating Mental Function

What kinds of stimulation work best for older people? Amazingly simple ones, as simple as taking a walk!

A study of long-term elderly state hospital patients provides an interesting insight. The subjects in this study had grown old in the hospital and they were deteriorated and vegetative, truly "the bottom of the barrel." They were divided into three groups. One group received a series of stimulating, new therapies such as occupational and recreational therapy and psychotherapy. A second group, used as "controls," continued as before in the custodial setting, inactive, with no responsibilities; they just sat about, were fed and slept. A third group was not involved in the therapy program but was taken for a half-hour walk daily to rule out any effects of physical exercise on the group who was receiving the therapies.

All were given tests of mental function before and after the study, and as expected, the therapy group outpaced the "control" group, who actually worsened with the passage of time. Not expected was the remarkable recovery of the group who simply took walks! They outpaced the therapy group by far. Not only did their mental functions improve significantly, but they began to speak up and assert themselves, much to the annoyance of some of the staff, who complained that they had become "management problems."

Was it the physical stimulation that did it? Only partly. They had reactivated important *basic decision centers* of the brain that had long been dormant—and the simple *act of walking* did it.

These people had not walked outside in years. They walked in long corridors and probably had not even looked from side to side for years. Think of the countless decisions that had to be made as they negotiated the paths outside the institution. As they bumped into each other and turned corners, they were *relearning* an automatic act, and apparently that kind of learning starts everything else going, too.

The lesson for us is this: the longer we live, the more necessary it is to *deautomatize* ourselves now and then: to pay attention to details we no longer are aware of. This sparks the mind and promotes concentration.

After all, isn't this what meditation is all about? First we are taught to "empty" our minds. Then we must concentrate on a leaf, a syllable, the tip of the nose, examining every detail, to heighten awareness. The simplest stimuli sharpen attention for everything else.

Certainly we need new experiences, new settings, and new relationships. But we need to be aware of them before we can benefit from them!

By the way, are you planning to walk for awareness? Next time, try paying attention to how you walk. Do you march *one*-two, *one*-two? Try *one*-two-three, *one*-two-three, *one*-two-three. You'll be pleasantly surprised.

More Myths about Learning

It is claimed that older people are harder to arouse, harder to motivate to take a test. Nothing could be further from the truth. One investigator measured the physiological responses of older people while they were being tested and discovered that they were too motivated. They were much more aroused than the younger people, which may be why they came out poorly in comparison: they tried too hard.

Of course, this is not due to aging. A young person who feels low on the totem pole will also be overly anxious to do well on a test. Fortunately, these high-arousal states are short-lived, and once the anxiety to do well is overcome by the older people through familiarization and a return of self-confidence, they do well.

Tests of learning capacity on older people invariably give mixed results, and for good reason. We are usually comparing the wrong groups: old with young instead of rich with poor, or educated with uneducated, healthy with sick, or foreign-born with native-born. For these are where the real causes of learning differences lie. People can perform on learning tests only to the degree that they have verbal ability; and they have verbal ability only to the degree that they have had health, wealth, security, good education, and good genes. It has nothing to do with age.

But there is also hope for "low-verbal" older people; trained in specific aids to learning, they will improve on tests.

Many of the myths of learning, along with the notion that older people are rigid, opinionated, and unable to learn new things, came about as a result of the first studies on aging, which were cross-sectional studies. They compared large groups of older people with large groups of younger ones.

In effect, they were comparing foreign-born, poorly educated immigrants with American-born youths who were reared, educated, and nourished in this land of plenty. In addition, most of the elderly people who were studied lived in institutions. What chance did they have on a test!

Fortunately, pioneering gerontologists like James Birren and Bernice Neugarten, followed by many others, revolutionized our concepts about aging by observing healthy, functioning older people living in their communities—and by using longitudinal studies which compare individuals with their own performances over their life-spans.

What did they find? That there were no significant changes in mental functioning during the normal aging process. Most of us, about 95 percent actually, live out our lives with no unusual breaks in functioning. When there are breaks, they are usually caused by other factors, such as emotional conflicts, environmental and social stresses, or physical problems such as deafness, blindness, and other disablements. And while their causes may not be preventable, these mental breakdowns are both preventable and reversible.

Even that old standby, memory loss does not hold up in longitudinal studies. There may be no loss of memory over the years; when there is, it may have nothing to do with age. All things being equal, there is no significant loss in basic memory function until after the age of 80—again, probably for reasons other than age.

Motor speed? Reaction time? Not nearly as bad as we have been led to believe. Reaction time can be improved with training and practice. So can motor speed, as anyone who has taken up swimming again after many years will attest. In any case, when there is a drop in these two areas, it is usually around that crucial sixty-fifth birthday, and it remains about the same until eighty (when most testing stops).

We now know that older people learn the way everybody else does, and they unlearn in the same way too: they unlearn from disuse of the skill, from frustration, and fear of failure. They learn by being rewarded for their learning and by experiencing a feeling of satisfaction. Above all, they learn from seeing a result.

What Is Relevant?

Older people, it appears, do not do as well as the younger on tests that require discriminating between the relevant and irrelevant. They tend to pay attention to details, thus missing the main point, or taking longer to solve the problem. However, at the same time they absorb more incidental information, which may come in handy, although perhaps not on that particular lab test.

Older people of today were trained to look at all

aspects of a situation; and their tendency to take in everything does not necessarily reflect an inability to ignore irrelevant details. It simply means that in their youth there weren't computers to do the work. Nor was there an impersonal organizationl structure they could pass the buck to. They had to do all the work, and they were responsible for the work they did.

So what may seem irrelvant to the young researcher may not be to older ex-workers whose life experiences taught them they better not miss a single detail, or else!

In any case, with a bit of briefing and a chance to get used to this new approach, older people usually improve, although they are probably never entirely comfortable with it. They certainly should not be labeled "inflexible" because they are overly cautious.

Intelligence Tests

James Birren, whose remarkable work has greatly changed the climate for those of us approaching middle and older age, discovered that among healthy people intelligence tests show little or no deterioration with age. This includes people in their seventies, eighties, and even nineties.

True, some people in the older age groups do show rather dramatic declines in intelligence, but they are the exception. Birren felt that if there were primary biological reasons for these declines in intelligence, they would show up in every individual and not just in some.

Given good health, there is little mental change up to age sixty-five and beyond, even on challenging tests of intelligence. Birren and most experts agree that health is far more important than age in determining the ability to maintain intelligence.

Age changes, when they do occur, may reflect changes in a person's mental set. A man of seventy will approach an intelligence test quite differently than he would have at the age of twenty.

In addition, older people have more "interference' in their thinking due to previous learning than younger people, for the simple reason they have learned so much more over their longer lifetimes. The retrieval mechanism (the ability to dig a fact out of your mind on demand) is slower in older people, probably because they have so much more material to sift through. Such "deficits" are simply the results of living—hardly the results of deterioration.

When people are tested against themselves in longitudinal studies, they are able to solve even complex problems of abstract reasoning with very much the same competence they had when they were younger. The trouble with most lab tests is that they reveal averages, not individual differences; on the average, older people may show declines in intelligence. As individuals, they usually do not.

A decline in intelligence, especially if it takes place at a crucial age, is usually related to the stresses of the particular period and not to the age of the person. In the 1960s many young people were led to believe that at age thirty, they would be over the hill. Believing this, many of them indeed did show signs of "decline" on tests. What happened was that they wound up with a bad case of "middle-age depression," though obviously these young people were not declining because of their age. Cultural trends made them feel old.

The "old-age crisis" can strike at any age, and when it does, our functioning declines, regardless of our ability or age. Scientific graphs of intelligence sometimes take a sharp dip at "crisis" birthdays, especially the sixty-fifth.

As we grow older, certain emotional states are inevitable, particularly depression. When a person is depressed, mental function is always affected. Fortunately for most of us, all this amounts to is "good and "bad" days, and we soon learn to pace ourselves accordingly, taking our ups and downs in stride. This is why the vast majority of older people weather the problems that come with living—without losing points on their intelligence tests.

The Mind Grows When You Do!

Unless you are stimulated, which involves a kind of challenge to the status quo, the mind stagnates. If you have been stagnating, you may have to start from the bottom up. Those mental hospital patients who took a daily half-hour walk outside the grounds got their minds working again better and faster than the ones who were given all the fancy "therapies."

The myth was that once the brain deteriorated it could not grow again. Not so. At the "Healing Brain" conference in 1980 in San Francisco, studies were presented that show that the brain develops, expands, and even heals itself after injury if there is stimulation and activity. Not only that, but according to neuro-psychologist Dr. Marian Diamond, there is actually a spurt of brain cell growth in older age that is comparable to the spurt of growth which occurs in youth. It is not known yet whether this increased brain capacity means "wisdom" or the potential for increased mental activity.

In either case, if there is no stimulation and outlet for action, the brain will atrophy from disuse. The potential of the older mind will be wasted. The tremendous movement to provide educational opportunities for older people (and their overwhelming acceptance of them) is perhaps the surest guarantee we have that the mind will have the chance to continue to "grow" all through life.

We already know that people who have not been educated show the greatest declines in mental function as they grow older, and we are now finding out that they also show the greatest improvement when they are exposed to education later in life. Education promotes attention. It also promotes the ability to rule out the irrelevant, which older people seem to have so much trouble with on tests. When you are learning something new (which is what education is all about), you are forced to ignore extraneous details in order to concentrate on the main point.

Education also forces one to communicate, organize thoughts, make different connections, and develop new approaches. When learning something new, you must start with basics; and when the mind acquires new building blocks, the results are bound to be good.

Love and Learning

Love makes learning a lot easier.

When somebody loves you, when you love yourself and have strong self-regard and self-respect, you can learn almost anything with ease. What the poets and the songs say aside, there is a scientific explanation for this. Love releases hormones and hormones release DNA (the memory part of the human cell), which in turn increases the function of the mind.

When you are warmed by the glow of approval, your own or someone else's, your brain produces chemicals that make you more alert and receptive. When nobody loves you and you have lost faith in yourself, your brain produces chemicals that contribute to being depressed and withdrawn.

This is true also of animals. In the laboratory, animals who are petted and talked to by researchers learn much faster than those who are ignored in their cages, and as a result may never learn at all.

A smile, a word, a touch works wonders. Although we may learn from our mistakes, studies show that we learn much better from our successes—that rewards are better than punishments.

However, it is also true that people who are geared

for success are willing to attempt more challenging tasks, whereas people who fear failure will avoid them and choose only those tasks they are sure they can do.

Such over-caution and fear of failure, which characterize the test performance of older people, are among the main reasons the tests themselves are invalid. In one study, the older subjects had to be urged to "take a guess" and "be a gambler" in order for the researchers to get any responses out of them!

Older people learn and respond most readily in non-pressured, open-ended situations. When circumstances become tighter, they may need emotional support to give them the self-confidence necessary to take "risks" and achieve success. This is true of young people as well; the difference is that emotional supports are much harder to come by as you age.

Ultimately, what we are talking about is the *libido*—the life force, the pleasure principle. This positive energy, with which nature endows us and which makes our activities pleasurable, may have become submerged with the passage of years; but it is still there.

Of course "old dogs" can learn new tricks. They may just have to practice up on a few old ones first!

Chapter Two

The Myth of Senility

"Nothing is at last sacred but the integrity of your own mind."

—Emerson

"Poor Aunt Harriet ..."

They had to take her away. Senile, you know, just not all there anymore."

We've all known an Aunt Harriet or Uncle George, relatives, friends, and sometimes parents who, growing older, seemed not to be playing with a full deck.

Until recently, any lack of mental functioning or peculiar behavior in a person over sixty was lumped under the term "senility," a catchall diagnosis reflecting more the confusion of the physcan than the state of the patient. What used to be called senility, and sometimes still is, was a series of unrelated symptoms believed to represent inevitable, irreversible deteriorative changes due to the aging process.

Today, senility is more often seen as a psychological breakdown in reaction to various crises of aging, and is not considered either irreversible or inevitable.

It took a long time for this point of view to develop however, although the facts have been known since the 1940s. At that time an important series of studies at Harvard University showed that there was not necessarily a relationship between hardening of the arteries of the brain and the actual functioning of the individual. People with quite extensive brain damage due to arteriosclerosis functioned well until they died—usually at a ripe old age and still working at their desks!

Others with perfectly intact brains were "senile" for years before they died.

"Good News about Senility!"

So reads a headline in *Modern Maturity*. The *Washington Post* proclaims, "Thousands Doomed by False Senility—Dementia Label Mistakenly Applied." Both articles have the same message: they are debunking the senility myth.

The "good news" is: "The latest medical and scientific knowledge can relieve one of humankind's greatest fears—the dread of senility, of loss of mind and memory." What is so often labeled "senility" is both preventable and curable.

"When people see an older person experiencing memory loss, however slight, or showing signs of irritability or confusion," the *Modern Maturity* article states, "their nearly automatic reaction is, 'Aha—senile!'"

The point is that any number of psychological and social stresses can bring about this kind of "senility." There are also many illnesses that can bring about temporary mental symptoms.

There is one major brain disease that results in senility. It is called Alzheimer's disease and possibly is a congenital disease like Down syndrome, or Mongolism.

But it affects less than 2 percent of elderly people and usually shows up in middle rather than old age. Ninety-eight percent of us need not worry about it.

What we should be worrying about, as the *Washington Post* article shows, is being *mislabeled* as "senile" and shipped off to a nursing home or mental institution without treatment! The *Post* reports that between 300,000 and 600,000 people labeled "senile" really suffer from a variety of other conditions which could be treated, if doctors recognized the true symptoms.

"Miracle Drugs Reverse Aging in Senile Patients"

No, this is not a tabloid headline; it is a serious report describing a group of new drugs—anticoagulants—which can reverse the aging process in certain senile patients. These anticoagulants allow the blood to flow freely to the brain, thus curing many of the symptoms of senility which previously may have led to a helpless, vegetative existence.

In a study at the University of California Medical School, at Irvine, anticoagulant drugs are used to treat seriously impaired elderly patients and have already had significant results in bowel and bladder control. With such regressed patients, this is an important first step towards improvement in other areas.

Another treatment being used successfully in mental breakdown in elderly people is oxygen therapy. Sometimes the results are quite dramatic, but improvement may be only temporary if there are underlying emotional conflicts. After all, senility can be a psychological defense, and people are not about to give it up if real life holds no value for them.

These new drugs and treatments mean that even that small percentage of seriously brain-damaged patients may now be helped. Other newer drugs, treatments, and nutritional studies are on the horizon, promising even more positive results. The attitude that, "They're old anyway, why bother doing anything about it?" is fast disappearing.

Want To Take the "Senility Test"?

Have someone else ask you the following questions very rapidly, and see how you do. More important, how does it make you *feel* to have to answer questions like these? Be sure not to peek now at the questions.

1. What is today's date?
2. What day of the week is it?
3. What is your phone number?
4. What is your address?
5. What did you have for dinner last night?
6. How old are you?
7. What is the date of your birth?
8. What should you do if you find an envelope in the street that is sealed, addressed, and has a new stamp on it?
9. Who is the president of the United States?
10. Who was the president before him?
11. Starting with number 1 and add 7 to each new number until you reach 36.

You answered them all—or maybe you had a little trouble with one or two. Anyway, it does not really matter unless you happen to be in an institution or a nursing home. In that case beware. A slip-up could affect your diagnosis and cause you a lot of trouble, especially if you're trying to get out of the darn place!

What Is Chronic Brain Syndrome?

You have heard it mentioned of course, usually when somebody's old aunt goes "bonkers." Chronic brain syndrome is what people have when they lose their memory, become confused, and don't know who or where they are—and when they are over age sixty-five. There are other names for it when one is under age sixty-five.

Old people who have chronic brain syndrome are often whisked away by those proverbial men in white coats to spend the remaining years of their lives in mental institutions or nursing homes.

But today, many psychiatrists take issue with the notion that chronic brain syndrome is the predominant disorder of old people. They believe that older people are subject to the same neuroses and psychoses as everybody else and that the symptoms of "chronic brain syndrome" are really the symptoms of a variety of other mental disorders which are overlooked.

Depression, a major mental illness of older people, is an example. It is often misdiagnosed as "chronic brain syndrome" and goes untreated. Indeed, if one were to treat the mental disorders that are lumped under "chronic brain syndrome"—such as depression, obsessive-compulsive neuroses, and paranoid psychoses—senility could well become almost extinct.

Physicians and families should also be aware that almost any physical illness may cause psychiatric symptoms in older people. They are more susceptible to "body poisons" resulting from a malfunctioning kidney or liver; they are also more likely to respond catastrophically to the stress of an illness, sometimes with "instant senility."

But their confusion and disorientation may be only temporary—if handled properly. If not, they may indeed become permanent and thus qualify the patient for the diagnosis, chronic brain syndrome.

Can the Brain Renew Itself?

Recently, since the development of modern scientific

methods for examining the brain, researchers have been making the surprising discovery that the brain can indeed renew itself in many ways.

Myth held that once there was injury to the brain, it was finished: the injured part could not regenerate itself as other organs of the body do.

An article in *Psychology* describes these extraordinary new findings. Brain injury does leave a scar. But new nerve fibers develop and grow like "fine branches" into the injured area—and the function that was lost returns. Not only that, other cells in the brain, which are believed to serve a restorative purpose, begin to multiply soon after a brain injury, and actually travel to the injured spot. They help to repair damage very much the way the blood cells do when they travel to an injury to help fight infection.

Now, scientists are even questioning the time-honored theory that the brain shrinks with age and that is why the mind deteriorates. New evidence indicates that we do not lose our brain cells with the years (except sometimes from disuse!) and that we can even grow new ones with stimulation. Most important, there is an increase in DNA, the memory part of every cell, with aging.

If the old man seems to be "losing his marbles," we better look for the cause somewhere besides the brain! In short, what we commonly call senility is not due to old age; nor is brain damage. It can happen to the young as well.

What we usually call "senility" is a late-appearing psychosis. Its causes are the same as those of any other psychosis. And its cures are the same.

Overwhelming stress, frustration, or anxiety—this will cause mental breakdown at any age. Add to that isolation, lack of stimulation, and a life without purpose; and the result is memory loss, confusion, disorientation, irrational behavior, and incontinence—which are the symptoms of serious mental breakdown at any age. Yes, even including incontinence.

The difference is that when a mental breakdown occurs in younger people it is called just that. In the older person, it is called senility.

Can the Senile Be Saved?

Of course. So don't panic when you hear "senility" or "chronic brain syndrome" in connection with someone you know. It is not an irreversible condition; there are treatments for it just as there are for other psychoses.

Senility can also be stopped before it starts. Watch for the danger signals of depression, insomnia, loss of appetite, mood changes, and irritability. Sometimes there are obsessive worries. These are warning signals of impending breakdown which may be overlooked as just signs of "growing old."

When these symptoms appear in young people, they are rarely overlooked. A young person who cannot eat or sleep, and who complains of poor concentration is quickly referred for help. We don't expect young people to be irritable and depressed.

What does one do if a mental breakdown has occurred? Is there some way to bring the person back again? There is a very simple therapeutic approach called *reality orientation* that is practiced in many hospitals and institutions in this country and others. But you don't have to be a professional to try it. It can be done—and should be done—by anyone who has contact with a senile person.

It is simply a matter of reorienting the senile person to time, place, and person—reminding the person again and again, of his or her name, the date, the time (including lunchtime, dinnertime, and so on) and of where the person is at a given moment.

This prevents patients from withdrawing and regressing. They are forced to be aware—whether they like it or not. Once aware of these basic realities, they are accessible to other forms of therapy which will help overcome the senile psychosis. These include various forms of psychotherapy, rehabilitation, and drug therapy which are used successfully with younger patients.

Simple Exercises to Do at Home

Grandma is a great-grandmother now, and she isn't what she used to be. Still, she is not a bother to anyone, sitting quietly in her room and taking care of her own needs. Even if she were a bother you would never consider placing her in a nursing home.

But you wish she would take more interest in what is going on around her. There is something you can do to stimulate her. It is simple, doesn't take much time, and even children can take turns doing it.

It's a 20-minute session of structured questions based on *categories,* which forces grandma to think while she is having what seems like a fairly ordinary conversation.

"Grandma, what were your favorite courses when you went to school?"

"Tell me a little bit about New York City" (or Duluth or wherever she lived).

"What sort of clothes do you like to wear in summer?"

"Tell me about some of the people in the family I never met."

These questions can be part of a game or a serious exercise.

"Name as many animals as you can."

"Name as many cities and towns as you can."

"Name as many things in this room as you can in five minutes."

"Name as many presidents of the United States as you can."

"Name as many foods starting with the letter *C* as you can."

In order for the exercises to be effective they must be done on a regular basis and not for less than twenty minutes at a time. There should be no prodding: grandma may have all the time she needs. Long pauses are okay, even no answers at all. It is important to sit quietly and be patient, and friendly for the full twenty minutes. Grandma will catch on soon enough, and as time passes, will enjoy her signs of improvement—as much as you will.

Scenes from "Senility"

A neatly dressed, attractive woman, much younger looking than her age of eighty-four is talking:

"I just don't know. It makes me so embarrassed and ashamed not to be what I was. I used to be a school teacher, you know. I did everything just right . . . now . . . I . . . I'm always so nauseous, so very nauseous . . . Can't you give me some medicine for this nausea?"

The woman looks and acts normal, except she keeps referring to her "nausea," disrupting all conversations with it. And she cannot be left alone because she wanders into the street and gets lost. Doctors find nothing wrong with her physically, no reason for the nausea and no brain condition to account for her confusion.

A few years ago, and even now in some places, she would have been given up as hopeless. Today, she is having psychotherapy, the "talking" treatment, and is beginning to improve. She refers less to her nausea, and instead speaks of "my disgust with myself."

Lately, too, she has begun to look for some antecedents for this feeling. "My stepfather disliked me. I remember that. Made me feel so stupid." "My daughter had a divorce, and then she had a nervous breakdown. Do you think I was failure as a mother?"

This woman's self-disgust was a long time coming. When it finally came to the surface, it came with such force it was converted into "senility." What is senility? In this case it was self-hatred and self-rejection.

A man of sixty-eight, always a friendly, happy, family man, is forced to retire, and shortly afterward he has a prostate operation. He becomes depressed, avoids seeing old friends and clings to his wife. The family tolerates this, friends accept it, attributing the changes in his personality, to retirement and the operation. They hope it will pass but manage to live their lives around him. He obliges by assuming the role of "shaky old man."

On the eve of his seventieth birthday, he suddenly accuses his wife of being a wicked stranger. They discuss this privately, and it passes. But the delusion returns frequently thereafter, eventually developing into a real drama—with a cast of characters who take over his living room. It is pretty obvious to all, except the man himself, that the "characters" are important people who in some way have cut him down, made him feel inferior: his boss, his father, even his son. When their "presence" sent him running in panic out of the house, the family decided something had to be done.

This man, too, had the "talking cure," and given a drug to help dispel his delusions. His insights were slow in coming: anger, guilt, and helplessness are difficult to accept. His "senility" was rage and revenge, feelings that this essentially gentle and loving man simply could not handle. Although he still cannot accept what happened to him, he has learned to recognize his delusions as delusions.

Sally is a lively, dynamic woman who has been married some forty years to a quiet, rather dull man. Until recently, she was involved in many activities, enjoyed her large circle of friends, and was an enthusiastic mother and grandmother. Lately she began to experience unusual physical weakness and started a round of visits to doctors which seemed unending. Some minor conditions were discovered and treated, but her complaints and the visits to the doctors continued.

One day she startled her husband and some friends by announcing that her eye doctor was "crazy about me." Since the doctor was at least thirty years her junior they assumed she was joking, but something about the way she said it made them uncomfortable.

Not long after that, she went into a profound panic after a sudden episode of incontinence. She rushed to the doctor as usual, and this time he recognized that a new element had been added. He suggested she see a psychologist.

She was immediately receptive to the idea and became a warm and eager participant in her own "talking cure." Her hearty, sensual nature was soon revealed in her spontaneous outpouring of feelings so long pent up and submerged in her inhibited marriage. She learned to value and redirect her strong sexual drives so that doctor-patient contact was no longer necessary.

Her "senility" was sexual frustration; her incontinence, a warning sign of regression to an infantile level of sensual satisfaction. She nipped it in the bud!

Why People Cling to the Senility Myth

Despite scientific evidence, and even their own experiences which disprove senility, many people still cling to the myth. Partly, this is due to the very natural tendency to expect the worst when your defenses are down. If you are sick, or in trouble, or even if a crucial birthday is looming (fifty, sixty, sixty-five, et cetera), any little sign of malfunction can activate the myth. The myth serves as a cop-out. "What the heck! There's nothing I can do about it anyway, once I'm senile."

"Senility" also serves an opposite purpose. When your defenses are up, and you are operating on all four cylinders, one of the last things you want to be reminded of is senile old age. It is such an extreme condition that it is easy to separate yourself from it: "Senility can't happen to me!" And, of course, the chances that it will are very slight indeed.

That's not where it ends, however. As we all know, when we create a "minority" group because of our own fears, the minority also becomes a target for our guilt and hostility. Senility becomes a receptacle for our negative, destructive feelings about aging, including our own feelings of hopelessness about our own old age. That may be why many studies continue to look for deterioration and overlook recovery. Pessimism can be a very subtle influence!

Let's face it—few of us can deal with growing old. When we do, we'd rather focus on the exceptions: those marvelous old people who continue to do things as if they were still young! They still play a pretty fast game of tennis (not including playing doubles—this is a sign of defeat), or still swim a daily twenty laps, or they take up disco dancing.

Our enthusiasm knows no bounds for these striving paragons. The fact that they can't let themselves relax means that *we* can—about age—at least for a while.

We are unimpressed by older people who use their time to travel, read, develop hobbies, and do the things they never had time to do before. Sometimes we are resentful and think of them as selfish, which is the way old people are supposed to become.

But older people who aim to please sure have their work cut out for them. Let the paragon slip up just once—let there be a moment of confusion or a single memory lapse—and the myth of senility stands by, ready and waiting. It may be annoying to forget a name at age thirty-five, but it's downright dangerous if you're past sixty-five!

"I'm Never Going to Let Myself Get Senile!"

The senility myth can serve as a form of self-discipline. It can keep you on your toes and it certainly makes sense to continue living with zest, providing we do not put out all that energy in order to avoid thoughts of dying. For eventually, repression of fears of aging and dying will consume all our energy, and we may end up "senile" anyway.

One way to avoid senility—and other less extreme problems of poor adjustment—is to *travel light* into older age, to leave behind excess burdens of anger, resentment, and hopeless longing. You may not be able to resolve these old conflicts (although many older people do, of course), but at least you can diminish them by becoming aware of them.

Most people are not afraid of death itself: they fear dying while life still owes them something. It's the bad debts that turn anger into anxiety and anxiety into senility.

While conflicts may not be resolvable, anger can always be "worked through,"—providing the greatest source of healthy energy a person has. Those who do not use up their energy store in the repression of anger will live much more fully.

How Angry Are You?

Answer yes, no, or sometimes:

1. Do you find yourself buying things you really don't want because the salesperson intimidated you?

2. Do you feel uncomfortable returning things to a store?

3. If your neighbor's TV is too loud, can you phone and ask him to lower it?

4. Do you have trouble making conversation in social gatherings?

5. Do you think others find you boring?

6. Do you find them boring?

7. Are you satisfied with your social life?

8. With your job?

9. With your family life?

10. Are you able to refuse a friend's request if necessary?

11. Are you able to make a request of a friend?

12. Can you criticize a friend?

13. Can you accept a compliment from a friend?

14. Would you rather swallow your anger than "waste" it by making a scene?

15. Do people push you around?

There is no score to this test. Your answers tell you something about yourself. If they indicate feelings of dissatisfaction with yourself or others, you are angry. Try to improve the situation you're angry about soon, but don't repress your feeling of anger. Remain aware of how you feel. Remember, you do not have to act on your feelings, and nobody can hear what you are thinking.

Chapter Three

Memory Loss May Be Good for You

"My enemy . . . I mean, my memory"
—A sixty-five year-old's slip of the tongue

Pursuit of Memory through Memory Loss

Suppose you're having trouble these days remembering names, places or past events. Let me reassure you that it's not because you are getting along in years, or your brain is failing you. Forgetting happens to younger people too.

Maybe your memory is trying to tell you something. It may be blocking out a word you want in order to draw your attention to something on its own priority list. And maybe you should listen to what your memory is trying to tell you, instead of wearing yourself out trying to remember the missing word.

The next time you cannot think of a name or words don't bore everybody with your searching. Just say, "Bill's brother, the one who lives in Minneapolis" or, "You know, the word that means those feelings you get

49

before something is going to happen" and continue your conversation. Later, when those elusive words are still bothering you, try the following. It is called "the *pursuit of memory through memory loss.*"

First, relax completely or do something that leaves you free to think, like taking the dog for a walk, and let your mind try to free associate to that missing word. Many different words and thoughts will come up, but not the one you are looking for. Spend a bit of time with each one, examining your feelings carefully as you do so. If an association makes you feel a bit tense, stick with it; now forget your original word and free associate from the one that has caused tension.

Soon, you will be facing memories and feelings that you hid away some time ago. Try not to push them back into your unconscious, try instead to deal with them. Remember, you probably won't be able to resolve anything, at least not right away. All that is asked is that you face the thoughts. By now they won't seem so terrible, anyway, and may even strike you as downright silly. You might wonder why you had to repress them in the first place.

Soon after this, your memory will present that missing word. Even if it does not, you won't care because you have given yourself a mini-analysis, and it did not cost a cent.

Test Yourself for Memory Loss

Look at the following words for three minutes and register them in your mind.

Column. Old. Moment. Numb. Spouse. Terrace. Operation. Apple. Friction. Death. Pepper. Mother. Camel. Dread. Will. Report.

Now check off the words you have memorized from the previous page on the following list.

camera	ghost	matter
train	old	column
meeting	daughter	plant
heaven	numb	moment
thread	spouse	heart
vision	terrace	operation
place	desk	carpenter
mother	auction	illness
pavement	report	supper
trouble	friction	apple
will	crutch	doctor
shadow	pepper	death
ugly	marriage	dread
camel		

If you failed to check off the following words, it means your emotions have interfered with your memory. This seems to happen more often as we grow older.

old	numb	spouse
operation	death	mother
dread	will	

Basic Memory Laws

No matter what you may have heard or experienced regarding loss of memory (or your mind) as you grow older, the fact is that the basic laws of memory are the same for everybody. All memory loss has a purpose which is usually unconscious and emotional.

The emotions block, distort, displace, and rework memory in people of all ages in much the same way, and for the same reasons. To put it simply, everyone tends to remember the pleasant and forget the unpleasant. Of course, what seems pleasant or unpleasant may vary for different people and may even vary for one person at different times. One forgets to do the wash, but remembers to keep a date for the movies, or remembers the wash, but forgets the dental appointment. Pleasant, as far as memory is concerned, simply means less painful.

It is the personal emotional significance of a particular event, whether it is threatening or comforting, which determines whether it will be remembered, and when and how it will be remembered.

Almost fifty years ago, F.C. Bartlett, a pioneer researcher in memory, proved that all memory tends to be altered to form a good gestalt, or psychological pattern which must not only be pleasing but must also fit the individual's past experience, feelings, and expectations. When we compare our memories with those of people who knew us in the past, we are often astounded by the scenarios which surround both our and their memories. If we are willing to be honest, we can see how self-serving and ego-protective these scenarios are.

However, even if a memory itself is unthreatening, a memory loss may occur if you are in a situation which is threatening. This is a major reason older people do not perform as well on memory tests as younger people. And even when no one else is testing them, older people are secretly testing their own memories, constantly judging themselves by what they forget rather than by what they remember. It is annoying to forget a name at thirty, but, it's a disaster at sixty.

Perhaps the greatest cause of memory loss in older people is that everyone else expects them to lose their memory and they are also sure that they will!

You Can't Remember What You Don't Register

The expectation that you will lose your memory as you get older is learned in early youth, and it influences memory and many other mental functions thereafter. It not only makes older people over-cautious, it even influences the kind of experiments that will be done on them. Few studies look for strengths in older people. How many of us knew that the biggest drop in memory function takes place between the thirties and forties? After age fifty, the decline is so gradual it never reaches statistical significance. If older people knew this, they would not be so cautious in learning new material.

In one study comparing older and younger people, the older group moved too slowly and their extreme caution in evaluating new material prevented them from responding to the test items in time. They lost out, of course, on this memory test, but it turned out that they had retained a great deal of "incidental" information, which was not scorable on the test.

This indicated a kind of global attention which may be a natural comcomitant of aging, learned from necessity and experience. The toll it takes of specific attention should not be labeled "memory loss."

In another study, a young group, a middle-aged group, and an elderly group were given a memory test and compared with each other. Each group was shown three sets of pictures: a contemporary set, showing a digital clock, dune buggy, computer card, and the like; a familiar set showing a baby carriage, telephone, et cetera; and an old-fashion group of pictures, including a spittoon and other vintage items.

Each picture was flashed on a screen, and the subjects identified the items as quickly as they could. The older people were faster at naming the vintage pictures; the younger people were faster on the contemporary set; and the middle-aged were somewhere in the middle. They were almost even in naming the familiar pictures.

Obviously, there is more to memory loss than memory.

When there is memory loss, it is important to ask what other losses this person has had. A job? Spouse? Status? Has the person been sick or moved recently? There is a strong suspicion that older people at times opt for memory loss rather than facing the real issues. It gives them a convenient "out," and it is the expected thing anyway.

It is interesting that some "senile" people do better on certain memory tests than normal older people. They may be able to repeat a series of digits with greater ease and fewer errors, and sometimes can do it backwards as well. Having "tuned out," their "senility" insulates them from anxiety—leaving them free to take a matter like remembering numbers in stride.

How "Screen Memories" Work for You

Pleasant memories are always more readily available to us than unpleasant memories, which may be why older people seem to dwell so often on a happier past—even if "happy" only means far enough back in time as to be no longer threatening. But this does not always work, and certain memories may continue to arouse anger or fear, no matter how far past they are. In this case a "screen memory" may be added for extra protection.

Screen memories are irrelevant, unthreatening memories which the mind obligingly substitutes for unpleasant memories that are trying to poke through the unconscious. Screen memories help block their passage while at the same time providing an outlet for the tension buildup which invariably accompanies the drive to remember.

When our defenses are down for whatever reason, emotional or physical, we begin to have all kinds of peculiar notions and sometimes might even act "crazy." This is because it is harder to control our unconscious during such times, and screen memories have come to the rescue. They may put strange ideas in our heads, but at least they keep those dangerous, repressed thoughts out. Screen memories are not necessarily pleasant, either; sometimes an old, unpleasant memory will be substituted for a more recent one simply because it is further away in time.

One seventy-year-old woman, who was slowly finding her way back from a profound memory disturbance of some two years duration, insisted that her last meeting with her son had been at her husband's funeral several years before. She "screened" out her most recent contact with him, when he had asked for, and she had refused, a loan of a large sum of money. Up to this point, she had been unable to remember anything at all about her husband, including his name.

Logically, the protective role of memory loss (or memory screening) should become more pronounced as one grows older, and it does. The longer one lives, the more things there are that are better forgotten. Even in the absence of any threat, it is necessary to forget more and more, simply to remain efficient. If one constantly remembered everything that ever happened, the result would be chaos. Could Mother Nature have meant us to have memory loss?

If we led less complicated lives, and had less to remember, would we have less memory loss? It would seem so, but that does not turn out to be the case: memory thrives on complications. There's an old adage which says, "If you want something done, ask a busy person to do it."

Studies show that the more educated, experienced, and involved we are, the better our memory in older age.

Memory thrives on novelty and stimulation, and especially on the *emotions*. That's right, the very emotions that can bollix up memory are also the key to remembering. Emotion opens up the memory block it may actually have caused in the first place!

But before there can be memory, there must have been motivation to pay attention. Motivation requires that emotional push we call interest, and interest requires the emotional reward of gratification.

There must also be emotion in order for a memory to be "registered," and every memory is deeply imbedded in its own emotional aura, or mood. That is why it is easier to recall something by first recapturing the feeling that accompanied it. And it explains why we sometimes remember everything about a person except his or her name.

As we know, we remember the same event quite differently when we are elated and when we are depressed. Elated, we block out memories we had when depressed, and vice versa. But either way we are in for trouble, because it is *unreleased* emotion which causes memory loss.

The body, gearing itself to act on an emotion—be it anger, love, or fear—produces adrenalin, other hormones and chemicals which must be released through some kind of action. If a person has enough outlets that excite and gratify, chances are that the tension buildup that causes memory loss will never occur. If this is not possible, then making the unconscious conscious is the next best thing.

The Return of the Repressed

Just as no memory is ever truly "lost"—but rather is misplaced—so no conflict is ever permanently repressed. When the unconscious eventually comes to light directly or indirectly, something has to give, and that something may be memory.

In the unconscious time, memory, and the emotions are intertwined; there is no concern for orderly sequence;

and past, present, and future are all the same. We know this from dreams, from sudden, vivid flashes of memory, and from those ongoing movies of the mind that confront us with some long-forgotten event and disrupt us at work or change our mood for the whole day.

Even in the ordinary course of daily living, it is a constant struggle simply to keep track of time. Where would we be without clocks, calendars, and the daily newspaper? It is even easier to forget the date when sick in the hospital, or on a vacation.

When there is a lapse in the sense of time, whether due to illness, accident, or anxiety, the mind—which cannot tolerate a blank—must fill in the gap. This substitute material is almost always of a wish-fulfillment nature and is dredged up from the unconscious.

In an extreme case, memory "loss" may occur like this: a father will clearly describe his daughter's wedding, list the guests, possibly even remember the cost. But he cannot tell whether it happened last year or twenty years ago. Consequently, he is not sure what year it is, or how old he is. Faced with this time lapse, he may improvise outrageously to fill in the gap. He may change his whole story to save face, claiming his daughter is a little girl, or does not exist at all, or is his wife. Then, panicked by what he hears himself saying, he feels forced to justify and defend his inconsistency and confusion. In his struggle to maintain a sense of time, any kind of time, he will adamantly insist that his illogic is logic and his unreality is reality.

But, you might object, this is not just memory loss. It is a mental breakdown due to an emotional conflict. You are correct. Not all emotional conflict leads to memory loss, of course, but there is rarely memory loss without emotional conflict. And in pathological aging, we see the end result of memory loss in mental breakdown.

Extreme forms of memory loss are rare; after all, only a very small percentage of older people ever become "senile." For the rest of us, it is only important to know that the unconscious breaks through more easily and more frequently as we grow older, interfering with the timing of our memories and causing confusion, anxiety, and sometimes lasting puzzlement. Above all, it is important not to panic and to simply wait out a transitory moment of memory loss—or to be more exact, memory disruption.

I think it bears repeating that at such times we should listen to what our memory is trying to tell us. This may require some effort in sorting and assembling thoughts and feelings which have become separated from each other, but it will pay off in the end. There is nothing to match the exhilaration of a liberating new insight into what has been long tolerated, or suffered as an established fact of aging.

Unclogging the Memory Machine

Normally, we make the necessary repairs to our memories as we go along. When things get bad, some of us go for memory-training courses. Repetition of what is to be remembered, practice at remembering, habits of attention and self-discipline, and various tricks of association all aid memory and concentration. In fact, just the decision to do something and doing it has a generally stimulating effect on memory.

Those who have some sensory handicap, visual or aural, must learn to compensate for the loss of cues and input. To repeat: *we cannot remember what we do not register.* And people with a hearing loss in the right ear have it even tougher, for it appears that what is heard through the right ear is better remembered than what is heard through the left.

But the *control* side of memory can be developed. The other side of memory, the personal-emotional component, derives from our very natures, our life experiences, and the selective forces inherent in us. This side of memory cannot be so easily controlled. We have to learn to be aware of it, to ride with it, and most important, to provide it with healthy outlets so that it does not take control of us.

During periods of poor concentration and forgetfulness, when the personal-emotional side of memory is in the ascendance, it is necessary to relax, pace oneself, and rest until the memory rush (which we experience as confusion) passes. This poses no problem when we are young: we tell our friends we were "really out of it" last week, that "I have to get my head together." We do not assume it is "old age" if we forget where the car is parked, or panic on a test. But we do attribute these to old age when we are older. Even if memory later improves, the doubts accumulate.

If a memory problem persists, few of us would think of looking for other causes besides "growing old." One youthful woman in her early sixties, married to a man considerably younger, came to the clinic where I was working because her "memory was going"—she could not find the words she wanted when she was talking. Convinced that she had had a stroke, although doctors assured her that she had not, she felt that her memory loss was a result of this.

The fact that she was completely fluent in group therapy and individual sessions did not convince her otherwise. Finally, after weeks of therapy and mounting group pressure, she confessed that her husband had been impotent for nine of their ten-years of marriage. She had been fulfilling herself by going to school, where her word-finding difficulty became more and more apparent, at least to her. She felt guilty and insecure about the sexual problem because of her own somewhat checkered past; she had never told her husband about it, but she was sure he suspected.

The group came enthusiastically to her rescue and she began to see the usefulness of her memory "loss" to avoid facing the real issues of her marriage. It was more difficult for her to confront feelings about her own aging, however, even though she had chosen the age-related symptoms of memory loss and stroke. While remaining insecure about their age difference, she and her husband took the constructive step of entering a sex-therapy program.

Forgetting is as emotional a process as remembering and involves the same kind of selective logic. The primary law of forgetting is, of course, that one tends to repress the threatening and to settle for the less threatening. If there is guilt, and there usually is, forgetting may also serve as a form of self-punishment, as in the case of the woman who forgot words, thus providing some release for built-up tension.

Shame, the "Forgotten" Emotion

Perhaps the most important element in selective forgetting is shame. In a memory experiment of many years ago, the participants memorized lists of words, some of which had obscene, other meanings, or sounded like "dirty words." In repeating the lists, some of the subjects used many tricks, often unconsciously, to avoid saying the shameful words. In some cases, the "bad" words were completely forgotten, or were mispronounced to disguise the naughty-sounding syllables. Instructions and corrections by the experimenters were repeatedly "misunderstood" by these subjects. Finally, when all else failed, they blurted out the words with obvious signs of embarrassment, blushing, and stammering.

Selective forgetting may be expected to occur whenever shame is involved—as in a group of elderly ex-drivers who blamed memory loss for having allowed their licenses to expire. They gave many reasons for forgetting to renew them, such as other things on their mind or travel out of the country. Few were aware of their unconscious shame of being "elderly" drivers or of their fear of failing the driving test. Most denied these feelings when asked about them, "Didn't bother me at all ... don't even miss it ...", and in fact they denied any unpleasant feelings at all at not being able to drive.

Yet the trauma of having to give up driving because of age has been shown to be a major life-crisis influencing many other aspects of adjustment. Nor does it seem to be entirely due to the very real inconvenience of being unable to drive in a world of wheels. Rather, studies show, it is the ego-disturbing implications of decrepit old age which seem to be represented in the loss of the driver's license. It can be more disturbing, apparently, than even the first bifocals or the first full set of dentures. It takes a lot of memory loss to get one past the "loss of driver's license" crisis!

Selective forgetting may be a factor in the appearance of certain physical symptoms. The role of repression in psychosomatic disease is well known; but when shame and guilt are involved an element of self-punishment is added to the symptoms.

A widowed mother, anxious to play a dominant role in her son's life, developed excruciating neuralgia which finally led to extended treatment in the hospital with which her son, a physician, was affiliated. This in turn led to her moving in with him and her daughter-in-law. Her pain continued to be punishing, but the mother was able to sustain it heroically, and completely "forgot" her many past difficulties with her son and his wife. She further denied any difficulties in her present arrangement, even though the family was compelled finally to enter into counseling sessions.

Some people contract the same illnesses their parents had, often at the same age. Unconscious memory and selective forgetting may be factors in death itself.

Living in the Past Is Good for the Present

Despite what you may have heard, reminiscing about the past, far from being a sign of old age, may actually keep you young! Studies show that people who think about the past a great deal are usually content, more active, and better adjusted in older age than those who put the past out of their minds. Those who can take the bad along with the good on their memory trips turn out to be the best adjusted of all. This is because they are able to deal consciously with negative feelings and do not have to resort to energy-consuming repression to ward off anxiety.

A very effective treatment for deteriorated old people who have been committed to institutions is called Old Times Therapy. It involves playing old records, singing old songs, showing movies of the good old days, and bringing out the family albums. However, this is not just a matter of reminding them of the past. It is a means of arousing emotions, which in turn *activate memory*. Despite the stereotype that old people "tune out" the present and live in the past, there are few senile people who can remember the past.

In many ways, confusion is healthy reminiscence gone wild. The father who drew a blank of his daughter's wedding would probably not have done so had he been able to confront his negative feelings honestly and deal with them. Instead, he blocked the memory drive and was forced to fill in the blank spaces in increasingly lunatic fashion.

Why Memory Lapses?

Why do people forget to turn off the gas or lock the door or leave the car keys in the trunk?

"Their mind was somewhere else," you say, and you are right. When one's thoughts are somewhere else, the first things to go are those automatic acts that do not require thinking. But why don't these automatic acts just go on automatically anyway?

Well, they usually do.

But when people have problems on their minds they also have accompanying emotions, past and present, which ordinarily are repressed in the unconscious. All the unconscious needs in order to find an outlet for repressed emotions is a break in the "conscious" controls. The automatic act which a person is scarcely conscious of doing offers such an opportunity, and the unconscious seizes it and uses it for its own disguised purposes.

What purposes can the unconscious have in making a person forget to turn off the gas? There are many answers, obvious and subtle, depending on the individuals, how much repressed anger they have, whom they are angry at, what their choices for revenge are, how guilty they feel, how much self-punishment they need, and how much they expect to have these "old age" lapses. Also, how much they fear such lapses plays a part.

A middle-aged daughter came for help about her aged mother, who would leave the gas on during the day while the daughter was at work. She was worried that her mother might be asphyxiated. In the course of consultation, the daughter revealed some serious problems related to her own aging, particularly her increasing deafness. She identified herself negatively with her helpless mother, and her mother resented the daughter's spoken and unspoken attitudes. Awareness of these unconscious feelings reduced anxiety in both of them. The mother left the gas on less frequently, and the daughter worried less when she did.

If this kind of thing is happening to you, try free associating the next time you let all the water boil away in your tea kettle. See what repressed feelings and thoughts you come up with. No, it will not be necessary to leave your job or divorce your spouse—but you may get some helpful insights into both, and you will remember to turn off the gas and take out the car keys next time.

Is this hard to believe? Well, in the old days it would have been. But we are living in an age of psychological sophistication, and we know about repression, the unconscious, conflict, and the different psychological hang-ups. It is just that we sometimes lose sight of our own. But a bit of serious free association, with clues from our memory lapse, is sometimes just enough to put us back on the track.

The important thing is not to accept a memory loss at its face value. If you are older and are expecting to lose your memory anyway, then maybe you should work on the expectancy rather than the memory loss itself.

Experimenters in a study of memory in rats were told that one group was bred to be dull and the other bright. Sure enough, their results proved that the bright rats remembered their way out of the maze much better than the others. The experimenters, who thought they were engaged in a study of genetics, did not know that the two groups of rats were actually of equal intelligence and that the study was to test the effects of expectance.

A Good Memory Makes the Unconscious Conscious

Of course, some older people are absentminded, at least as much so as some younger people. If both groups periodically brushed up on their automatic acts, we might do away with absentmindedness altogether.

Even people who are relatively conflict-free are in danger of a takeover by the unconscious when their minds wander during an automatic act. That is why it may be a good idea to develop the habit of observing oneself from time to time in the act of starting the car or leaving the house (check for car keys, wallet, et cetera).

The habit of alertness will pay off if there are any unconscious motives lurking about, and you will be able to beat yourself at your own game.

Obviously, the purpose of such an exercise is not to make you perform automatic acts more efficiently; it may even have a temporarily opposite effect. The purpose is to strengthen *consciousness,* thus preventing the intrusion of the unconscious in any situation, including automatic acts.

More important, memory is always aided by the conscious will to remember. (When this does not seem to be true, we probably are at cross purposes with ourselves.) In studies on memory, people who are rewarded with money or recognition of some kind, do better than those who are not, regardless of age. In other words, age seems to make no difference when people are consciously motivated to remember. Nor does it when people are unconsciously motivated to forget.

Conscious awareness of unconscious conflict should make memory improve. Perhaps you already proved this to yourself after taking the memory test on page 50. A person of any age who deals with conflicts as they arise usually has a good memory. When there is unresolved conflict, the first thing to go is memory, no matter how young the person is. Memory loss is the major symptom in mental breakdown at any age.

Does a good memory guarantee that a person will be conflict-free insofar as this is possible? It depends on what is meant by "good memory. If it means the ability to rattle off figures and dates, it may not. This kind of memory, which is the goal of some memory training courses, may actually be a wall preventing the recognition of inner feeling and conflict. Some people who cannot remember where or who they are may be a whiz at remembering telephone numbers—any telephone number.

But if what is meant by good memory is the ability

to recall an event in its entirety, including negative, shameful feelings surrounding it, then memory can indeed make a person conflict-free.

How can one do this when the basic law of memory is to forget what is unpleasant and to remember what is pleasant? It is difficult, and for some people impossible. Self-awareness must be developed, and one must keep working at it. The natural tendency is for memory to change to fit the need, not the reality. When a person's defenses are down, memory loss comes naturally. But for an aware person, the loss will only be temporary. The habit of self-awareness (impossible without self-acceptance) will help prevent panic, which is the biggest cause of permanent memory loss.

Fortunately for most people, facing oneself becomes easier as one grows older. Experience and wisdom accrue, time and the mellowing process minimize old angers and frustrations. Some people will always lose their memory, of course. And it will become more obvious as they grow older.

But they will not lose their memory *because they are older!*

A Guide to Your Unconscious

Do your own psychobiography. It's a favorite exercise in group therapy and other kinds of know-yourself sessions. Your responses to the following questions will be absorbing and revealing. It does not matter how little or how much you write. Everyone sets their own limits on self-knowledge automatically—but the act of writing it down has a liberating effect. Good for you!

1. What were you like as a child? Any special talents? Difficulties?

2. Describe your parents and your relationship with each of them.

3. Write about your brothers and sisters (if any) and how you got along with them.

4. What is the earliest experience you can remember? Describe it in detail. Also your reactions to it now.

5. What other life experiences stand out in your memory? Describe them even if they *seem* unimportant now.

6. Do you have a recurrent dream? Describe it, and any other recent dreams you can remember.

7. Evaluate your physical condition. How have illnesses and other physical difficulties you have had affected your way of life? Your point of view?

8. What do you like best about yourself now?

9. What do you like least about yourself now?

10. If you could live your life over what changes would you make?

11. If you had three wishes *now* what would they be?

12. On a scale of 1 to 10, 5 being "so-so," how would you rate your life-satisfaction level?

Chapter Four

Problem Parents of Middle-Aged Children And Vice Versa

"How come you're getting a divorce after forty five years?"
"We wanted to wait until the children got theirs!"

What Happened to Good Old Dad and Mom?

Today's children still get furious at aging parents, but they're furious because they don't act like aging parents.

It used to be said that old people don't have problems until they *become* the problem. Well, today they solve their problems before they can become a burden to their children.

Although the media, social workers, and do-gooders tend to focus on the sick and homeless, or the destructive effects on children and grandchildren when an old parent invades their nest, the fact is that the vast majority of aging parents are breathing a deep sigh of relief and settling down to enjoy life. . .

. . . Somewhere a good distance away from the children!

The Alienation Myth

Just as the study of aging has been distorted by the myths, so the situation between children and aging parents has been distorted—especially by the myth of alienation.

To start with the "good old days," when the old parent supposedly filled an important role in the family—gerontologist Ethel Shanas reminds us that very few people survived into old age then. Those who did helped about the house and did not threaten anybody. They were tolerated.

The role of the old person as the dispenser of wisdom and the inspiration of grandchildren is true, of course, in some cases. But for the most part it is a literary creation, a banner waved for a cause—and a favorite theme of TV commercials. Modern older people are not all that eager to dispense their wisdom—they'd rather enjoy the fruits of it. And if they are going to babysit they seem to prefer to do it for strangers—for a fee.

And, as Shanas puts it, "They even have the temerity to live alone!"

Ninety-five percent of all persons over age sixty-five, including those who live to be past one-hundred, continue living in the community. Less than eighteen percent live with their children, or their children with them.

Does this mean the rest are alienated? Far from it. Most live near their children and visit frequently. But today's older generation places a high value on having their own households; they want independence and privacy as much as their children do.

Since the economic situation for both old and young has improved in the last twenty years (improved compared to what it was, not what it should be for all citizens), this has become largely possible for both generations.

But what about those horror pictures we are always being shown of abandoned old people wasting away in nursing homes? Surely, they are not a myth? Surely, they are alienated?

No, they are not a myth. Yes, they are alienated. Almost one of every eight people over the age of eighty is institutionalized. But most of them are *not* problem parents; most are single or do not have children. It is those who are either bedridden or housebound because of illness and who have no family to take care of them, who end up in nursing homes.

Even they are a tiny minority. Most of the very old can now be maintained in their own homes, and they prefer it, adapting as they go along, and deciding for themselves when the time has come to give it up.

Younger people (this includes anyone below 80) may find these facts discomforting even though they represent such a small percentage. But isn't it good to know that ninety-five percent of us can be our own person until the very end?

Why Do We Need the Alienation Myth?

An interesting question. We shudder at the sight of the elderly silhouetted against the windows of lonely apartments, looking at the world going by.

We weep along with the reporter who recently wrote a heartrending story about lonely old people in Miami Beach who just sit and gaze at the ocean—completely overlooking the fact that most are refugees from the inner cities and are delighted to sit safely and drink in the beauty of sun and water.

Why doesn't someone *ask* them if they are lonely? And what about the thousands of other older people who live in Miami Beach who do not have time to sit on the beach? Are they lonely, too? Any more so than their children are?

The real question, of course, is why the old person sitting on the bench or at the window is called "lonely" while a young person in the same position is "dreaming," "meditating," "observing."

The answer is that we have fewer and fewer places to put our guilt. As Karl Menninger pointed out in his book, *Whatever Became of Sin?*, most of the bad things we used to be punished for now go unpunished, if not unnoticed. Adultery is an amusingly quaint notion of times gone by. Murderers make deals in the courts. Crime and sin have been objectified—nobody is held personally responsible.

But individuals want to feel responsible, even if society says everything is okay. They have to do something with their guilt, whether it's their own or society's.

What better way than to flagellate themselves through the voice of the media about the traditional, time-honored sin of abandoning the old? Confession is good for the soul. Political activists also need a good cause. It's the old person, who refuses to fit into the alienation myth, who is the problem—whether a parent or not!

It Makes Good Dollar Sense . . .

. . . to maintain the alienation myth. Ethel Shanas observes: "there has been a special emphasis on programs to meet the needs of these alienated, aged people who, in keeping with the myth, are supposed to be the majority of the aged. The truly isolated old person, despite his or her prominence in the media, is a rarity. . ."

Shanas comments on the powerful bureaucracies organized to fill the needs of the old person they have conjured up in the "age of the social worker," and to provide "services" that are rarely used by the elderly and their families, even if they are aware of them.

What are these "services"? How do they fit the needs of the elderly? A recent survey points up startling discrepancies.

A group of service providers and a group of elderly persons were each given a list of eighteen "needs" to rank in order of importance. There was little agreement between the two.

In almost every instance, the service providers followed the alienation myth while the elderly themselves contradicted it. For example, the providers put "housing" near the top of their list, and the elderly placed it last. The elderly wanted "personal safety," "consumer protection," and "home repair," while the providers went for "leisure-time activities."

They only came close to agreement on "income." The elderly placed it first, the providers second. (They ranked health care first.) But while the elderly put tax relief in second place, the providers (wary of a reduction in funding?) put it far down, in tenth place.

The survey also produced the sad news that trained service providers were inaccurate in determining the needs of the elderly. It was suggested that they had developed "tunnel vision," and the recommendation was that the elderly themselves should make the crucial decisions as to what their needs are.

It all boils down, as Carroll L. Estes explains in her book, *The Aging Enterprise,* to economic bureaucracies creating their own realities "in the interest of the aging," and deciding what are to be the real "problems." Neither Estes nor anyone else would suggest that government ignore the elderly—least of all the elderly themselves, who are accomplished activists in their own right.

But they want to be the ones who decide what their problems are.

The Problem Parent Who Is "Put Away"

Despite the mythical aspects of alienation of the elderly and the companion theme, abandonment, the hard truth remains that 5 percent of the older population, especially those over eighty, are in nursing homes and other institutions.

Even though it is only a small percentage who are institutionalized, and most of them are *not* parents, many older people and their middle-aged children live in secret dread of this eventuality.

Even those who are not fearful think it is because they are "lucky" or because their family is "different." They cannot relax with the knowledge that ninety-five times out of a hundred, an older person may expect to live out life at home—neither alienated nor abandoned.

Think of what this myth does to family relationships! It turns parents into "good guys," children into "bad guys," and puts everybody on the defensive. Parents and children may even share a mutual paranoia.

One helpless, guilt-ridden daughter who couldn't bear to see her mother waste away in a "home" (which the mother herself had insisted on going to because she did not want to be a "burden"), came for help.

"I just can't stand her being there. But she was so unhappy when she was with us. She didn't like the food, and the children annoyed her with their noise. Yet she doesn't eat in the nursing home either, and I doubt she'll live out the year."

"Are you thinking of taking her back?"

"I'd *like* to, but the only place that's quiet is in the basement, the den. How can I put my mother in a basement?"

"Why not ask her? Only call it the den, why say basement?"

"She simply refuses to eat my cooking, she'll starve."

"You say she does here anyway."

"True. I'll ask her. Let it be her decision."

Indeed, let it be.

When decisions like this are made for parents, even when the decisions are in their favor, the parents resent it. This is a natural reaction—it makes the parents feel powerless and the only power that remains to them is bucking the decision.

They may come up with a better solution of their own.

One eighty-year-old woman who suffered a stroke was placed in a rehabilitation hospital and saved from "senility" by the constant vigilance of a dedicated staff. As she began to recover some function, the problem of future placement loomed. No way would she become a burden to her son! But she was not averse to sharing a house with her nephew, paying half the expenses, and providing her own equipment. She preferred the location, her nephew was alone and could use the financial help.

Although she had run the gamut of feelings from abject dependency to paranoid grandiosity while in the hospital, her eventual decision was a sound one. Her son had enough sense to trust it.

Most Parents Stay Put

Today, it is rare for children to place their aging parents in a nursing home.

When they do, it is because the situation has become extremely disruptive, the parent so psychotic, that normal family life is no longer possible. Even at this stage there are alternatives, as indicated in other chapters, but many "kindly" family physicians do not seem to know them.

With all good intentions, they advise children to put mom or dad in a nursing home, and the children in desperation may act on the advice. But the physician should also warn the children of the lifelong effects on *them* after putting their parents out—because no matter how much reassurance they receive, children always feel they have committed a dastardly act. It is a burden they will carry every after, unless they are forewarned.

Their guilt is irrational, because they did their best. But they may need counseling and even psychotherapy to keep that guilt within bounds and prevent its destructive effects later on.

There are very few middle-aged children who, having placed their parents in a nursing home, do not suffer severe after-effects in crisis periods during their own old age. There are many maladjustments, disguised in various ways, that have at the core the guilt of that act. It is a vicious circle.

Fortunately the numbers of people involved are growing smaller and smaller.

And where it has occurred, "putting the old parent away" has often had a beneficial result—on the grandchildren. New evidence is proving that younger people of today, horrified because of what they know about nursing homes from the media, are taking a stand against the "warehousing of older people."

The Gray Panthers, a powerful activist and lobbying group for the rights of the elderly, is actually a coalition of young and old activists. The field of aging itself is being invaded by young students whose ideas and contributions are not only refreshing but practical and effective.

In my own experience over the past year, three grandchildren have taken over the board and care of their grandparents when it was not feasible for their own parents to do so. In the vast majority of cases, however, when elderly parents become incapacitated, they tend to stay put—sometimes with their own brothers and sisters.

With the lifespan increasing on the average, more brothers and sisters are surviving, and there is a general tendency for sisters to move in with brothers when they are widowed, and vice versa. New combinations of surviving relatives are making "moving in" with the children less necessary.

An interesting sidelight to emerge from one recent study is that young people have more positive attitudes toward the disabled than do people who are middle-aged. This finding came as rather a surprise, since it was expected that the middle-aged would have more sympathy and tolerance because of their own first-hand experiences with ill health.

The study suggests that during the period when the middle-aged are working out their own feelings about aging, it is perhaps better for the old to be with the old, or the young.

In "retirement" communities, which are becoming increasingly popular, the average age is often the middle seventies. The middle-aged children of these retirees, who may be retired themselves, prefer "adult" communities where the average age is somewhat lower (but not much) because they fear the stigma of retirement. Their attitude has some justification—"retirement" is too broad a term for people who have only retired from work, not from life. But their real reason is fear of identification with the next phase of life—their own aging.

That is why shrewd developers have created both "retirement" and "adult" communities. And grandchildren happily visit both and have a fine time on the tennis courts, golf course and in the swimming pool.

Problem Parents and the Middle-Age Crisis

In order to have an aging-parent problem, you have to be an aging child, or worse than that, you yourself are in the throes of your middle-age crisis. If you can wing it through middle-age without a crisis, the chances are that your parent will, too.

As anyone who has ever been in family therapy knows, the family in stress needs a scapegoat. As insoluble conflicts mount, the tensions need to be siphoned off on someone. That someone is usually the one with the least power.

The children of problem parents are usually in their fifties and sixties, and they may be problem parents in their own right. They are facing or experiencing retirement, physical changes, reduced income, or maybe disappointment in their own children. It is an age when widowhood and other catastrophes strike—when major life adjustments are required.

Middle-aged children and their parents are part of the same life stage, and their experiences, both inner and outer, are identical. But the last thing the middle-aged child wants to do is identify with an aged parent—while the parent has never given up identification with the child.

The middle-age child is fighting old age. The parent uses this as a weapon; and the one who is less vulnerable, and therefore more powerful, will win.

It could be either one.

It is very rarely "easy street" between older parents and middle-aged children. Those who get along fine think that they are exceptions to the rule. Parents and middle-aged children who get along usually live apart, and the parents are usually active, involved, youthful types who present an acceptable role model for the children.

On the other hand, the opposite is also true. Children sometimes resent the parent who is obviously enjoying life—particularly when they themselves might not be. The parents, for their part, are made to feel guiltier and guiltier—it's very much a "shoe on the other foot" situation.

The "swinging" older parent and sullen middle-aged child may be a specific problem of our times. Those in their sixties and seventies today have gone through a remarkable series of strengthening life experiences, having not only survived depressions and wars, but also having made such gains for their own survival as Social Security and Medicare; and most of all, they have come into a new social environment that is favorable to them.

Their thirty-five- and forty-five-year-old children may *not* have developed the inner strength of their parents. Many who were born late in the depression years have remained dependent to some degree. Some even return home to the parental bosom because things are too tough for them.

Problems of the Parents

A group of seventy-year-olds met regularly for "consciousness-raising" sessions in a Miami Beach retirement hotel. The issues were as follows:

Was it wrong of them to dip into the grandchildren's college fund for a trip to Hawaii with the group?

How to tell a daughter *not* to send the grandchildren down for the Easter holidays because grandma was all booked up for the week.

How to tell a daughter not to send the grandchildren down because grandma has a boyfriend living in.

And so forth. Parents are rebelling, but not without guilt. Many of the issues brought up in psychotherapy groups are fraught with guilt over using up the inheritance, indulging oneself, abandoning the *children!* But parents are getting there.

They are weathering the jealousy of their own daughters as they go dancing and dining. Some are not, though. One pleasure-oriented widow finally had to give up and take her daughter in to live with her. But she didn't do so until she was sure the boyfriend with whom she had broken up was not coming back.

Older parents are in fact doing most of the things they were doing as younger parents, with some adjustments here and there, as the ranks of suitable "partners" thin out.

Middle-aged children will have to search out new scapegoats—or hopefully, they will work through their middle-age crises instead.

Why Parents Become Problems

If things are going so great for older people, how come *any* of them become problems?

Because even though older people have been able to recapture most of the props of good living these days (and that includes work, play, romance, travel, and education—all of which are currently available to those who want it) the most important element of all is missing.

That element is power. The experience that is truly unique to older age is loss of power. It takes some getting used to, and some never make it.

Older people call it, euphemistically, "being needed." When asked what is worst about being old, they invariably answer, "Not being needed anymore." Young people believe this, too.

Older people, as we know, are also terrified of being dependent and unable to take care of themselves. This is the young person's greatest fear of aging also.

So if everybody wants to be needed and nobody wants to be dependent—who will do the needing?

And, since all relationships involve transactions, isn't this really a matter of who will have power over whom? What happens to the one who doesn't have the bargaining power?

Plenty! Loss of power is probably a major factor in all problems between middle-aged children and their parents.

It may be why older people are gravitating towards peer-group communities and self-help programs, which put them back in the driver's seat. Among themselves, responsible for themselves, their bargaining powers are put to use again.

But what about those who stay home?

It is not unusual for old parents who are given "the best of care" in their children's homes to become more and more unmanageable until they must be placed in a daycare center—where they blossom into friendly, active participants. And back again to their old selves when they come home at night.

One grandmother nearly had a nervous breakdown when her daughter hired a nurse to take care of the baby.

"Why are you so upset?"

"Because now that nurse is taking complete care of the baby."

"Well, is that what you wanted to do?"

"No, but I was willing to sit two nights a week and take him every other weekend. Now they don't need me at all. They say, "Mom, just come and enjoy him. You won't have to do anything.""

But this woman wanted to be *needed*—on her own terms, that is. Of course she was "unreasonable." She didn't realize that she was no longer in the same position of power as when she was younger. Her alternatives were now limited, though her children's were not. So in her mind, it was a question of "put up or shut up." What a bind—for both her and her children.

It is interesting that even though men are hit hard by the loss of power in older age, they are rarely referred to as "burdens" by their children.

Mothers are seen as problems, are the ones who are most often regarded as "senile," by their middle-aged children. Fathers with the same symptoms are more willingly tolerated.

This is because children expect parents to be perfect—especially mothers and it is difficult for them to accept human frailty in their mothers. As we will see, "wayward" mothers are the ones who usually end up in the nursing home.

Mothers and Daughters

Perhaps things are tough for mothers partly because it is the daughter who usually takes care of the aging parent. But the seeds of trouble are present to begin with in that complicated, multidimensional relationship about which we know so little.

The mother-daughter relationship is still so sacrosanct that even researchers hesitate to go too deeply into the nitty-gritty. When they do, the mothers and daughters are afraid to read about it!

We are told, and believe, that mothers tend to prefer their sons, that they tend to be more judgmental and critical of their daughters. How true this all is doesn't really matter. Daughters grow up believing it, and the rest is history.

Some part of the trouble is the inevitable identification of mother with daughter. The negative feelings each has towards herself, and each other, surface and clash when the two are locked together in later life.

Sons take it more in stride in those far fewer cases where mothers live with them. They seem more able to separate themselves both physically and emotionally from their parents—and also experience less guilt about them. They are more realistic and more readily accept the fact that it is not within their power to make the parent truly happy. (It is impossible for a person to be "happy" in a position of dependency and powerlessness, but many daughters insist upon it and feel martyred when their parents don't comply.)

Men seem to regard economic responsibility as their main duty toward parents (even if this only means using their power of attorney to sign checks for them). Women, on the other hand, usually become emotionally involved with the parent. This includes wives whose husbands leave the emotional well-being of their mothers to them. No wonder it is easy to slip into the martyr role when tending an old parent: the daughter, or daughter-in-law, is likely to be damned whatever she does and damned whatever she doesn't do. The son, on the sideline, comes out smelling like a rose.

Battle of the Bank Account

Even in the best of families, the internal bookkeeping begins as the parents grow older. Consciously, or not, expenditures are evaluated in terms of "Is it worth it?" and "Does it pay at this stage?" Undeniably, money plays an important part in the difficulties that exist between parents and children. Of course, poor people are exempt from this problem, at least when it comes to questions of inheritance. But many still have difficult decisions with respect to the care and maintenance of their parents.

This is particularly true when an aged parent becomes sick, and the unconscious (or quickly repressed) hope persists that the parent will pass away before all the money is spent.

In fairness, many parents share this hope. The "living will" has become a popular document among those who do not wish to waste time and money on the tubes and appliances that will keep them alive for months after they are actually "dead."

But wouldn't it be wonderful if money never had to rear its ugly head? Then families could continue their usual relationships and avoid the inevitable guilt that accompanies the "inheritance blues."

Well, believe it or not, it's happening. *Modern Maturity,* reports that "more Oldsters Are Now Disinheriting Children." It is a new trend in wills known as "benevolent disinheritance." It seems that more and more older parents are cutting their children out of their wills in favor of friends or neighbors, the magazine reports. Parents who disinherit their offspring feel they have amply provided for them during their lives, that their grown children are financially secure and do not need help, and that a trusted friend or neighbor could use the money more.

"With more older people living in retirement communities or in situations where they are out of contact with their children for long periods, observers feel the trend is likely to continue."

Long live power to parents! Now children can sleep easy for the rest of their lives.

Chapter Five

Those Golden Anniversary Blues!

"I married you for better or worse, but not for lunch..."

Popular saying

"Grow Old Along with Me...

"... The best is yet to be." sang poet Robert Browning to his love, Elizabeth Barrett Browning. But Elizabeth, six years older than Robert, died when she was fifty-five while Robert lived on for almost thirty more years.

Perhaps it is just as well that Robert did not have to learn from experience that longer is not necessarily better when it comes to marriage. Researcher Judy Todd recently made headlines with her interviews of couples who were married for fifty years. The subject turned out to be unhappiness. What made them unhappy fifty years ago was still making them unhappy fifty years later!

Why did they stay married for fifty years? Well, for them marriage was important, not happiness. They saw marriage as a challenge, an obstacle course, a test of survival ability. They survived the depression, war, the marriage: "Here we are, two souls surviving in a world of distress. We made it."

They were lucky. Many long-married couples do not make it. Oh, they stay married all right. (Although younger couples with similar problems are usually counseled to get a divorce.) But practically every problem they have in aging is related to a basic problem of their marriage.

Marriage fifty years ago was not fun, at the center of everybody's life was the Great Depression. In the early stages of the marriage, most people worked long hours, the husband trying to scrape up a living, the wife trying to make do at home. Vacations were mostly unheard of.

Women in those years craved emotion and affection; men were taught to be cold and unemotional, and were disappointing. Intimacy as we know it today was rare. "Happiness" meant power, which is why most husbands felt in retrospect that they were happy in their marriages. They were decision-makers, they earned the money and decided how it was to be spent.

And they were the heroes—protectors of women and providers for children. Yes, they agreed in interviews, there may have been something missing but they didn't know what it was.

But the wives were bitter. They remembered the ploys they had devised to get what they wanted—direct requests were unheard of. "I wouldn't say anything, I would just look sad," said one wife.

What finally saved these women? Believe it or not, their husbands' retirements! Because their roles changed—from powerless to powerful. Not surprisingly, men of this era (and this type of marriage) felt worthless when they were no longer wage-earners, and they were more than willing to resign their at-home duties.

The wives learned to drive, began signing the checks, and soon were making all the important decisions.

The research produced at least one optimistic finding: the happier couples were those whose marriages had a more modern appearance, and in which the sex roles were more equalized. The men were more attentive and emotional and *shared* their power; they shared interest in the home and children. Husband and wife were a team.

The First Twenty Years Are the Toughest

Divorce after twenty years is not so uncommon these days, it's only after thirty years that eyebrows begin to be raised. But still, not many marriages break up after twenty years. Few couples even think of coming for marital counseling at that point; they simply swallow hard and figure it's not going to get any worse.

As a rule, the marriage does stay the same—which can be bad enough.

Seventy-eight "typical" Chicago couples interviewed after twenty years of marriage were rated as to the degree of approval or disapproval they felt towards their spouses. The results were astonishing: over half showed no approval at all of the spouse. Where there was approval, or for that matter clear-cut disapproval, it was a mutual feeling in only half of the cases. Most husbands approved of their wives, unaware of the wives' disapproval—and vice versa.

Talk of lack of awareness—of alienation! Yet these marriages moved along in appropriate fashion at least up to the twenty-year mark.

When couples approved of each other it had nothing to do with whether they were "well-mated" according to the personality tests and interest ratings each was given. "Approval" was related to social conformity, conventional attitudes, moderate political views, and to the fact that husband and wife were of the same religion.

As for disapproval, wives working at nonprofessional jobs shared a mutual dissatisfaction with their husbands. Career women, however, generally claimed to approve of their husbands, blissfully unaware apparently that their husbands disapproved of them.

Some of us may be thinking, well, it figures. Working wives are usually overworked and resentful; career wives make husbands feel inferior. But it seems it isn't that simple. Not all working wives are resentful, and many husbands are proud of their career-women-wives.

Power underlies the problems: who has it, how it is used, how it is misused. Power, particularly the loss of it, will be referred to again and again in this book. Loss of power, at least in the author's opinion, may well turn out to be the root of all evils in aging.

It certainly seems to be at the root of marital evils. For even when husband and wife are compatible, and approved of each other, the study showed, in the family where the children held the power, the marriage eventually went bad.

The 70-Year "Itch"

Marriages that stagnate after twenty years sometimes break up after forty years, or when one of the couple approaches the seventieth birthday. The repercussions and reverberations can be profound. One such momentous break-up rated a two-page feature story in the *Los Angeles Times,* written not by the jilted wife (she adjusted nicely to the flight of the husband) but by the outraged daughter.

It came as a total shock to her that after thirty-six years of marriage, her parents should separate in their late sixties, with all the children fully grown and gone—just when they should relax finally and enjoy each other's company.

But it seems that dad, after commuting sixty miles a day for thirty years, couldn't manage retirement. And mom, who had been dreading his retirement, found his presence and his "meddling" even worse than her expectations.

They hung in there for awhile, but then dad took up jogging and health foods and began using Grecian Formula, and soon the "other woman" popped up. They got a divorce, and dad married her.

Mom was amazed. "Can you believe it?" she asked. "I never thought I would be in this situation."

Their daughter was numb. None of her efforts had worked, even though her parents held off the divorce for a few months at her request and saw a marriage counselor. After the divorce, the remaining family unit stayed intact: mother is content with her own apartment and the visits of children and grandchildren. The daughter, who had therapy for several months, no longer has crying jags. For her, the pain is reduced, although the memory of it is still there.

The main difference is that she regards her father as a "non-person." But was he ever really more than that?

In the old days, marriages did not go on for so long. With the lifespan extending and with personality "growth" a real possibility even into old age, more people are finding it harder to settle for that walk into the twilight together—especially with a spouse you can just about tolerate.

Age seventy is beginning to match age fifty as a turning point in marriage. And it's not just the men who walk out. A surprising number of women do, too—usually when a long-time, secret, lover's wife dies and the path opens up to a new, much-awaited life.

If there is a difference between fifty and seventy, it's that at seventy one does not seek newer and greener pastures. A new marriage usually consummates an established love relationship that perhaps should have become marriage in the first place. For people of seventy today there are fewer restrictions, just as for every other age group, and it is just as hard to stick with a marriage that has soured. The wayward father of the *Times* article married an old high-school sweetheart, his first love.

Senile Breakdowns in Too-Long Marriages

The seventy-year "itch" doesn't always end in romance, however. In fact, it is more likely to end in senility—for one partner. We rarely hear of both spouses of the same marriage becoming senile. It is usually one or the other, or to be more precise, it is usually one who has been more *done to* than the other.

People need out, sometimes desperately, of a too-long marriage for a variety of reasons, and often with disastrous results. Marital problems are probably as much a cause of mental breakdown in the elderly as anything else.

But the theories of "senility" don't even mention marital problems as a cause. If marital problems are mentioned at all, they are usually seen as the result of senility, as when a husband no longer recognizes his wife and insists she is a stranger.

Disengagement theory claims that older people voluntarily withdraw from social and emotional stimulation, both for their own good and society's ("youth must be served"). Thus, it is "normal" for the aging to detach themselves gradually, almost as preparation for death. But the theory does not explain why in a marriage it is usually only one spouse who disengages while the other is still raring to go.

Activity theory, the opposite of disengagement, states that older people benefit from continued involvement and participation in society. Most evidence upholds this. "Well-adjusted" older people remain active; and successful marriages usually find both spouses busy and involved. But even activity theory does not tell us why a successful fifty-year marriage may suddenly sour.

And chances are, the affected spouse can't explain either. The reasons are invariably unconscious, longstanding, and better left unsaid—since there are other ways to settle such an issue.

Who's the Boss Now?

Sally and Henry R., both in their early seventies and retired, have been married over fifty years. They worked side by side in a little stationery store they owned, and despite brutally long hours, Sally also took care of the house, cooked, and raised the children.

It was a dreary marriage, as the children recall. They saw neither parent very much. When she was with them, Sally complained about Henry's attentions to women who came into the store and about his habit of taking off and going to the races while she stayed behind to work.

Ten years ago, Henry became blind. The children were terribly concerned for both parents, but they needn't have been. Sally ran the store singlehandedly for seven more years and saved enough to buy a small apartment in Florida (over Henry's objections).

They live there now. Sally swims, plays bingo, and has lots of friends. She takes good care of Henry, who is at home most of the time, and she arranges for sitters when she goes away. Sally also has a boyfriend, but Henry does not know about this; neither do the children, who have never ceased to be amazed at Sally's "get-up-and-go."

They are glad that she is not letting Henry's further deterioration prevent her from enjoying life. Even the doctors do not understand why he took such a turn for the worse when they moved to Florida. They had expected the opposite.

Obviously, existing theories of senility are not sufficient to explain the complicated dynamics of Sally and Henry and thousands of couples like them.

But there is an economic theory that does. It is called Exchange Theory. Social-gerontologist, James J. Dowd has aptly applied it to marital relationships that go sour.

Power Exchange in a Marriage

In any relationship, according to the exchange theory, individuals will always try to increase rewards while at the same time reducing costs by various maneuvers. A relationship can be called profitable only as long as it is more rewarding than it is costly.

But in every relationship one of the participants will value the rewards more than the other. At this point, *power* enters the relationship: the one who needs the rewards less has power over the one who needs the rewards more—and enjoys a power advantage.

What is the reward for the powerful one? The compliance of the less powerful one and the reward of being boss. What is the reward for the powerless one? The use of the power resources of the other: protection, shelter, prestige, support and status, all of which are benefits that usually accrue to wives.

What happens when the powerful one loses power? The power balance shifts. In aging, people generally —and men especially—lose their power advantage. The same thing happens in the long-lasting marriage. The dethroned one has to look for new sources of power—or assume the compliant role.

Where does the power come from? It is always there: one of the mates is always more powerful than the other in some areas. Thus, there can always be an exchange of rewards and a balance of power in the relationship. When one or the other can no longer "pay their way," when one has nothing to offer, there is no longer a balance of power and that person is in trouble.

Four Ways to Fight Back

Gerontolgist Dowd refers to four possible balancing operations which I will apply to marital situations to illustrate the steps older people take to reestablish their power—and which is sometimes confused with "senility."

Withdrawal: The powerless can withdraw their needs. "I don't care for what you can give me anymore, therefore I am no longer in your power." They then become depressed, apathetic, stubborn, noncommunicative. They may even bring illness and death upon themselves.

Extension of the Power Network: The powerless may take up outside activities, develop new skills, gain new status. This is healthy. Or, they may develop grandiose fantasies along those lines, together with suspicion and hostility towards others who are "out to get me." This is paranoid.

Reemergence of Status: Those who are down are helped up by being honored again for former skills. Their wisdom is sought once more, they are respected for what they were. This always happens in a good marriage; for instance, when the husband retires. It didn't with Sally and Henry—revenge was too sweet.

Form a New Coalition. A few years ago, when older people saw their rights being taken away from them, they formed a coalition with a group of young activists and started the Gray Panther movement. This was good strategy for renewing power.

When a husband, believed mentally incompetent, was threatened with institutionalization by his wife, he formed a coalition with gangster elements in the community and lost all his and her money in a bankrupt bar and grill. He emerged poor—but feeling powerful.

"In Sickness and Health"

In a good marriage, in any good-relationship, dependency is not a disgrace. Power means the power to *give*. Reward is the well-being of the other. Many long-lasting marriages are like that and often have to withstand the well-intentioned but misguided efforts of family and friends to maintain their own balance.

One loving couple had their lives disrupted when the husband began to deteriorate rapidly after retirement, becoming senile. Dependency was never a problem with them, because he had always been dependent upon her, and she enjoyed taking care of him. Perhaps his deterioration was due to some late-blooming brain disease, or perhaps it was a sudden displaced assertion of long-repressed power needs of his own. In any event, his wife took it in stride, continued to care for him, and enjoyed it.

The family physician and their children advised institutionalization. She had her own health to consider, they told her.

So off he went to a nursing home and pined away until he became comatose. She pined too, until her blood pressure reached a dangerous peak. Finally, unable to bear seeing him in such a state, and without consulting anyone, she packed him up and took him home.

There she cared for him, cooed over him, and kept him clean. He began to smile again and even managed a few words now and then, revealing the man who was still there. Both bloomed in the relationship that had always been natural for them. He died after several years, at peace and in his own bed. She mourned him a long time and then spent her remaining years engaged in many activities surrounded by friends and family. When she died several years later, she was very old and very much at peace.

This happens more often than one would think. But of course there is also the opposite situation.

"Til Death Do Us Part?"

With some couples, the last thing they want is to stay together until death. They panic at the mere possibility of sickness—often in the disguise of a marital problem.

"I simply cannot take his meddling any more. He's at my heels everywhere, criticising, getting in the way. And the children blame me! They say he was always this way. Well, if he was then I've had enough. Is it so terrible to want a separation at this age?"

Real problem: husband has severe hardening of the arteries and was warned by a physician that a stroke was possible. His wife is panicking at the prospect; she wants out before it's too late.

Even when there is honest self-awareness, facing a future with a chronically ill spouse is difficult, sometimes even disabling to the well one. Many stress-related illnesses occur in men and women who are faced with this problem. The dilemma is a real one and must be dealt with in its every aspect.

It isn't enough for the physician and the children to put their okay on a nursing home placement, since this can be even more emotionally stressful for the well one. The problem has to be worked through, just the way grief has to be worked through, and that takes time. It may end with a nursing home placement, but the remaining spouse must be made aware of his or her guilt, fears of retaliation, and all the negative feelings that have been repressed over the long marriage, just as one must be after death of a spouse.

The scenarios that some spouses force themselves to go through before placement is both pathetic and destructive to both. Children are often the least helpful, urging a hedonistic attitude (you have your own life to live) when that isn't the problem at all.

It isn't a matter of living one's own life. It's a matter of *identification*. Will this happen to me? Can I accept it if it does? Are there alternatives? Can I live with this guilt? What kind of children are these anyway? And so on.

Selling the Sick Spouse Down the River

Nobody consciously wants to do it. The very thought is usually deeply repressed and did not necessarily arise when the spouse first became sick. It started long before in what invariably was a miserable marriage and was really a cry for separation.

But separation was not possible for whatever reason, and the marriage lumbers on until sickness hits. Even then the sickness is not the issue. It is having to nurse the sick one that puts the plan into operation.

And what a convoluted project it can be! Such detours and smokescreens—doctors and family can be fooled until the final scene. Even the main actors, the spouses, can never be sure of the ending.

Mr. W. brought Mrs. W. to the clinic with an intractable cough that had been diagnosed as "psychosomatic." There was nothing wrong with her physically: she needed psychotherapy. The only problem was that the cough was so constant there was no possibility of conducting the talking treatment.

Mr. W. who seemed attentive and concerned enough did his best to help, but he had difficulty communicating since he had recently had an operation for throat cancer. However, he did provide the information that his wife's cough started at the time of his operation.

Aha! *Identification,* everybody thought. Mrs. W. got her illness by suggestion. Very well, they would use suggestion to get her out of it. Mrs. W. happily agreed to try hypnosis and enjoyed almost instant recovery.

But it didn't end there. Shortly after, Mrs. W. came to the clinic herself and asked to see a marriage counselor. Several sessions later, after she had unburdened herself of thirty-years' worth of marital wrongs and resentments, she was able to face the reality of his illness and its effect on her.

In a few more sessions, she felt she had resolved the issue, claiming to be aware of her revulsion and fears of his having recurrences of the cancer, and to be in control of them. She also knew that she could not leave him— she felt too sorry for him—and in any case, all she would have was a small Social Security allowance, not enough to live on. She went home.

The counselor had misgivings. This did not seem like the end to her, but she had no idea what the next act would be. It was almost six months before she found out.

Mrs. W. rushed into the clinic one morning in a state of high agitation and required sedation. It seems her husband had taken to beating her. She never knew when an attack would come and had gone to live with a niece. Well, the previous night he came to the niece's house and was so threatening they had to call the police, who placed him in a mental hospital. Should she or should she not have him committed?

Mr. W. solved the problem by voluntarily committing himself for treatment. He was acutely depressed and had spells of uncontrollable agitation. He said he was no longer a "complete man" and that he knew his wife wanted to get rid of him. After treatment, he was willing to enter marital counseling sessions together with his wife. Some weeks later they came to a reasonable adjustment of their finances and agreed on a divorce. They both recognized that their's had never been much of a marriage, and neither had much to gain by continuing it. Mrs. W. got out of it with sufficient funds and a clear conscience.

Even in the absence of a specific problem or fear, many husbands and wives take a long look at the next phase of marriage when the seventieth birthday approaches. Again, there are many unconscious factors at work, and sometimes the only outward signs are depression, sudden irritability, and unaccustomed impulses.

When repressed feelings are worked through and become conscious, husbands are more willing, as a rule, to settle for things as they are. As we said before, they are not averse to giving up a bit of the male prerogative —such as driving the car, balancing the checkbook, and the like. If their anger and resentment remain unconscious, however, they may make a fetish out of the car or the checkbook, driving their wives to distraction in the process.

Women, on the other hand, tend to compensate for frustration with fantasy and may have to be pushed to face reality. The reality is that after age seventy, the ratio approaches two women to one man (who is usually married), so that the chances for a fresh try at romance are very slight indeed. The life of a lone woman, while considerably improved over past years, is still by no means enviable.

Wanted: Someone to Care For

Not all spouses want to get rid of the sick one—far from it. Most are willing to fulfill their marriage vow, "in sickness and health," if only their well-intentioned advisors would leave them alone.

Some people actually need a sick spouse to feel worthwhile. This applies especially to husbands and wives who may have collected a few guilts over the years and find this a way of expiating for past sins while enjoying the admiration of others for their kindness.

They are the bane of every professional worker who is trying to do something about curing "senility." Every clinic has cases of spouses bringing senile partners for counseling on how to manage at home. It's a beautiful thing to see—but, beware of how far you go to "help" them.

Clients on the verge of recovery are often unaccountably withdrawn from treatment. Various lame excuses are given, and some outright lies: "She's getting worse," when she's obviously getting better. But the real reasons are never touched on, because recovery means trouble! First, the senile spouse on the road to recovery will be getting all the repressed rage and hurt out of his or her system. Second, the recovered spouse will be a new person, someone to contend with, someone who will surely upset the applecart.

Even in less drastic situations, there are benefits to be gained from caring for a sick or senile spouse at home. The spouse who is the caretaker gains a sense of health from the other's dependency. In fact, a sense of well-being may stem from the sickness of the other, even when the caretaker has real problems. By remaining active, independent and, above all, responsible for the welfare of another, a person may indeed ward off many illnesses that would otherwise strike.

What about the one who is being taken care of? Well, if one really is dependent and unable to manage, being cared for at home by a willing spouse is certainly the preferable alternative. But if one is being manipulated into dependency to feed the unconscious power strivings of a spouse, or to help ward off a spouse's fears of illness and death, then the position is not so comfortable. Then, there is only one way of restoring the balance of power—revenge. This is done with selective behaviors and symptoms that can make life a misery for the caretaker.

Of course, most of these maneuvers are unconscious on the parts of both spouses: no self-respecting couple would admit to such ulterior motives. But if they could bring themselves to face them (in counseling), then many golden anniversaries could indeed be cause for celebration.

Trouble Starts in the "Empty Nest"

The period after the children leave home has always been one of the most trying times of all for older couples. Nowadays, the "empty nest" period starts earlier and lasts longer than ever before. It puts marriage to a real test.

For a long time preceding the departure of the children, the couple had been relating to each other as parents. Now they must face each other as people, and sometimes they do not like what they see. Without trying to salvage the marriage, many turn to separation and divorce, following the trend of the times.

But this may lead to other woes. Apart from the fact that new partners are not easily available, younger people, and society itself do not have the same tolerance for such marital foibles among the older generation as they do for the younger. Reactions to late-life divorce may range from disapproval and shock to outright ridicule. Nowhere does "ageism" hit harder.

Older couples do well to cancel out the emotional debts accrued over their long marriage, and to focus on another range of mutual interests such as: maintaining a good income flow, retaining social status, working at good health, and continuing family and friendship relationships.

Effective use of leisure time is perhaps the most important new activity. No doubt each spouse will have diverging interests by this time, and this can be all to the good. The main reason many older couples stay together happily is because each spouse does his or her "own thing," in a kind of marital singlehood.

What's for Lunch, Mom?

It's dad, not the kids, who's asking.

As any wife will tell you, one of the worst things about retirement is the menus. Nobody ever bothered with breakfast before, and dinner used to be fun. But *lunch?*

One can learn to manage the three-meal-a-day grind, and retirement isn't what it used to be either. These days, it can be fun.

To begin with, older people aren't what they used to be: they can be fun. Second, they are only retiring from work, not from life. There are lots of things to do, and many retired couples are doing them—alone or together —including going back to work.

A great deal has been written about the retirement crisis, and it would be impossible to cover it all here. In any case, the older generation is changing so rapidly that what has been written quickly becomes obsolete.

But there are two important points to be made. First, retirement is a very new, twentieth-century phenomenon. Second, it may disappear as suddenly as it came. The retirement age has already been raised to age seventy, mandatory retirement at any age may soon be legislated out of existence.

If it is, it may well be the wives who complain. In many cases, they urge their husbands to retire, not only to fill the empty nest, but also to have someone to do things with during empty hours.

If trouble starts after retirement, it is usually due to the marital relationship itself, and more specifically, to a power imbalance. A man not only earned a salary while working, he also earned approval, respect, and self-esteem. It takes a while to find new sources for the latter three. If a wife assumes the leadership role (as many do) at this critical time while a husband's defenses are down, the die is cast.

The husband has no recourse but to resort to compliance, and the golden anniversary blues begin. Then, the wife begins to push harder to get a reaction from him. The husband withdraws more, and a "senility" pattern may set in. As aging expert Dowd remarks about retirement and the decline of power, "Over the years, as the scenario has been repeated countless times, the process has become routinized . . . legitimated." The withdrawal behavior of the retiree is not surprising, it is *expected*. But it is erroneously attributed to retirement, when retirement is only the straw that breaks the camel's back.

Restoration of self-esteem should start at home in the family, and dependency should be discouraged. "Why in the world are you asking me about the income tax return? You've been handling it ever since we were married! You know your way around the balance sheets. You tell me! And while we're on the subject, the children want you to continue doing theirs too."

They Had to be Doing Something Right

They've been married fifty years, staying together through thick and thin. They raised nice children; the grandchildren adore them. Neither has broken down—yet. That's the bright side of the golden anniversary blues.

Something can be done with this marriage. It can be revived and may even work better now in a different form. The goal is to *individualize* the spouses. Each should feel one's power as an individual—and should extend the same privilege to the spouse.

It happens automatically when opportunities for activities and the development of new interests are available. Retirement villages and adult communities are probably doing more to save the long marriage than anything else. Senior citizen centers are not so effective possibly because they are too controlled and directed.

In addition, it is essential that one be in control of one's own decisions. Individuality cannot be developed without freedom of choice. In other words, as each spouse becomes his or her own "person" once again—or perhaps for the first time—and values himself or herself and the other for it, the couple may well stay together "til death do us part."

Chapter Six

Dealing With Depression in Everyday Life

A man wrapped up in himself makes a very small bundle."

Benjamin Franklin

Depression—The Road to Nowhere

There are probably as many forms of depression as there are people, but all depressions have one thing in common. They turn a person away from the world—they lead nowhere.

Depression narrows one's range of activities—a depressed person does less and less.

Depression narrows the range of emotions. Contrary to popular belief, depression does not mean sadness; it means emptiness, and the depressed person is devoid of feeling.

Depression destroys relationships, because the depressed person withdraws from others even while needing them desperately for support—in fact, in order to stay alive. But the depressed person has nothing to give to a relationship.

Yes, the person who is wrapped up in himself "makes a very small bundle" indeed. But don't underestimate the power of that small bundle. Depressed people may not feel anything, but they certainly make themselves felt. Nobody likes to be with a depressed person, but just try and get away!

Depression—A Natural State

Nobody is immune to depression, although some people may have better defenses against it than others. It is a natural condition, a basic mood, a universal experience.

According to the Freudians, it is our first experience. Some believe that the very act of birth has in it the seeds of depression and may set the pattern for all later depression. It is claimed that even in normal child-rearing, the infant experiences depression with each pang of hunger and each absence of the mother, no matter how brief. But fortunately, the child soon learns to trust in her return. Infants in hospitals used to pine away until they were dangerously close to death. Once this was recognized as "infantile depression," steps were taken to provide "mothering" and the babies survived.

Whether or not the basic pattern of depression is set in infancy, it is quite true that the severely depressed do become "infantile" in their behavior. Like infants, they become demanding, impatient, and totally self-preoccupied. Other people exist only to the degree that they can fulfill the needs of the depressed. Like deprived infants, they are quick to despair and may not even recognize a helping hand when it is extended.

This is a natural state? No, of course not. It is an extreme result of a natural predisposition all of us have, and we can relate to it even if we have never experienced it. Depression is a basic condition in all our lives; our adjustment to life depends on our ability to conquer it.

This may seem like a "depressing" statement in itself, but it really isn't. Conquering depression means that it is no longer a danger to the individual. But one must be aware of it and able to recognize it in order to conquer it. Just as accepting death liberates one to enjoy life, so by conquering depression one is liberated to enjoy the other great universal mood—elation.

The Many "Masks" of Depression

"Me, depressed? Why I'm busy every minute. I don't let a minute go by without having something planned. I don't go to sleep at night— I collapse! No, sir. I'm not depressed. I don't have time to feel anything."

"Depressed? It's a miracle I'm not depressed. What with all the sickness I've had lately. I tell you it's been one thing after another. I must have gone to every doctor in town. The last one had the nerve to say I was a hypochondriac, can you believe it? No, I'm not depressed —just angry."

Depression.

The reason there are so many forms of depression is that there are so many factors contributing to it, so many different emotions, reactions, deceptions. There's rage, fear, loneliness, restlessness, obsessiveness, compulsiveness, the gamut of human responses.

But the very core of depression *is loss of self-esteem,* a sense of worthlessness. That is why it can be so hard to cure the depressed. They feel unworthy of rescue.

Loved Back to Health

Unfortunately, the only sure cure for depression, that most unlovable of conditions, is love. Pure, undemanding, unselfish love that is willing to give without question and without hope of return. The technical term for this kind of love is "narcissistic supplies." It is the kind of love mothers give infants who can only experience "love" insofar as it provides satisfaction of their needs. Infants, purely selfish in the beginning, knowing only themselves, are narcissistic.

The same is true of the seriously depressed person who has regressed to an infantile emotional level. The depressed need narcissistic supplies as much as the infant does, and it is almost impossible to fulfill their demands. Few people want to either. It is one thing to love an infant or small child back to health but quite another to extend the same kind of selfless devotion to adults—particularly since they probably have already turned off friends and family by negative behavior during the developing phase of the depression.

Even if some diehards remain willing to dedicate themselves to their recovery, chances are the depressed won't accept their efforts. Depression is not only an illness, it is also a way of life. In order to recover, the depressed person may have to start all over again. That takes a lot of doing—and it may be easier to remain depressed.

In such extreme cases, professional help is essential; otherwise, many innocent people may be sacrificed to the bottomless pit of the depressive's needs. It is much better to learn to detect the early signs of depression and to do something while it is still possible. Even better is to become acquainted with situations that typically breed depression, so that depression can be anticipated and prevented.

Probably no other human condition has been investigated as thoroughly as depression. The news is not all bad either. There are many effective cures, although the most effective cure is probably the knowledge about depression that is being disseminated in the press, in literature, theater, and through self-help efforts.

The do-it-yourself approach to curing depression is feasible, because it is based on self-knowledge that is available to everyone, and because it is a condition that is widely shared.

A Test to See If You Are Depressed

The *Beck Depression Inventory** is a questionnaire you can answer to learn if you are depressed, and to what degree. It should be answered before you read further in this chapter, or the score may not be valid. This highly regarded test of depression is used widely by professionals.

A. (Sadness)

0   I do not feel sad.

1   I feel blue or sad.

2a I am blue or sad all the time and I can't snap out of it.

2b I am so sad or unhappy that it is quite painful.

3   I am so sad or unhappy that I can't stand it.

C. (Sense of Failure)

0   I do not feel like a failure.

1   I feel I have failed more than the average person.

2a I feel I have accomplished very little that is worthwhile or that means anything.

2b As I look back on my life all I can see is a lot of failure.

3   I feel I am a a complete failure as a person (parent, spouse).

B. (Pessimism)

0   I am not particularly pessimistic or discouraged about the future.

1   I feel discouraged about the future.

2a I feel I have nothing to look forward to.

2b I feel that I won't ever get over my troubles.

3   I feel that the future is hopeless and that things cannot improve.

D. (Dissatisfaction)

0   I am not particularly dissatisfied.

1   I feel bored most of the time.

2a I don't enjoy things the way I used to.

2b I don't get satisfaction out of anything any more.

3   I am dissatisfied with everything.

* The author wishes to thank Aaron T. Beck, MD, for granting permission to reprint the Beck Depression Inventory.

E. (Guilt)

0   I don't feel particularly guilty.

1   I feel bad or unworthy a good part of the time.

2a I feel quite guilty.

2b I feel bad or unworthy practically all the time now.

3   I feel as though I am very bad or worthless.

G. (Self-Dislike)

0   I don't feel disappointed in myself.

1a I am disappointed in myself.

1b I don't like myself.

2   I am disgusted with myself.

3   I hate myself.

I. (Suicidal Ideas)

0   I don't have any thoughts of harming myself.

1   I have thoughts of harming myself, but I would not carry them out.

2a I feel I would be better off dead.

2b I feel my family would be better off if I were dead.

3a I have definite plans about committing suicide.

3b I would kill myself if I could.

F. (Expectation of Punishment)

0   I don't feel I am being punished.

1   I have a feeling that something bad may happen to me.

2   I feel I am being punished or will be punished.

3a I feel I deserve to be punished.

3b I want to be punished.

H. (Self-Accusations)

0   I don't feel I am worse than anybody else.

1   I am critical of myself for my weaknesses or mistakes.

2   I blame myself for my faults.

3   I blame myself for everything that happens.

J. (Crying)

0   I don't cry any more than usual.

1   I cry more than I used to.

2   I cry all the time now. I can't stop it.

3   I used to be able to cry, but now I can't cry at all even though I want to.

K. (Irritability)

0   I am no more irritated than I ever am.

1   I get annoyed or irritated more easily than I used to.

2   I feel irritated all the time.

3   I don't get irritated at all at things that used to irritate me.

M. (Indecisiveness)

0   I make decisions about as well as ever.

1   I try to put off making decisions.

2   I have great difficulty in making decisions.

3   I can't make any decisions at all anymore.

O. (Work Retardation)

0   I can work as well as before.

1a   It takes extra effort to get started doing something.

1b   I don't work as well as I used to.

2   I have to push myself very hard to do anything.

3   I can't do any work at all.

L. (Social Withdrawal)

0   I have not lost interest in other people.

1   I am less interested in other people now than I used to be.

2   I have lost most of my interest in other people and have little feeling for them.

3   I have lost all my interest in other people and don't care about them at all.

N. (Body Image Change)

0   I don't feel I look any worse than I used to.

1   I am worried that I am looking old or unattractive.

2   I feel that there are permanent changes in my appearance, and they make me look unattractive.

3   I feel that I am ugly or repulsive-looking.

P. (Insomnia)

0   I can sleep as well as usual.

1   I wake up more tired in the morning than I used to.

2   I wake up 2–3 hours earlier than usual and find it hard to get back to sleep.

3   I wake up early every day and can't get more than 5 hours sleep.

Q. (Fatigability)

0   I don't get any more tired than usual.

1   I get tired more easily than I used to.

2   I get tired from doing nothing.

3   I get too tired to do anything.

S. (Weight Loss)

0   I haven't lost much weight.

1   I have lost more than 5 pounds.

2   I have lost more than 10 pounds.

3   I have lost more than 15 pounds.

U. (Loss of Libido)

0   I have not noticed any recent change in my interest in sex.

1   I am less interested in sex than I used to be.

2   I am much less interested in sex now.

3   I have lost interest in sex completely.

R. (Anorexia)

0   My appetite is not worse than usual.

1   My appetite is not as good as it used to be.

2   My appetite is much worse now.

3   I have no appetite at all.

T. (Somatic Preoccupation)

0   I am no more concerned about my health than usual.

1   I am concerned about aches and pains or upset stomach or constipation.

2   I am so concerned with how I feel or what I feel that it's hard to think of much else.

3   I am completely absorbed in what I feel.

Now find your score by adding up the numbers you circled under each item. If you circled more than one number under a particular item, add just the higher number. For instance, if under Q (fatigability) you circled both (0) "I don't get any more tired than usual" and (2) "I get tired from doing nothing," then add 2 points to your score.

If your score is between 0 and 4, you're in good shape as far as depression is concerned. Even though you may have some doubts about your state of mind and your capacity to cope, depression is not your particular problem. If, however, you are convinced that you are depressed regardless of a good score on this test, then it may not be tapping your particular form or depression. Or this may be an unusually good day for you. The fact that you *think* you're depressed is more important than your test score, and you might want to discuss your feelings with a professional.

A score of 5 to 7 is usually indicative of mild depression. A score of 8 to 15 indicates a moderate degree of depression. If your score is over 16, there may be potentially serious depression and you should consider seeking help.

You will notice that depression is comprised of a great many feelings that most of us have experienced at one time or another, although perhaps not all at once. There is nothing "crazy" about depression, nothing unfamiliar. Very few of us are strangers to depression.

Symptoms of Depression

Depression comes with a great variety of symptoms. To make matters worse, some symptoms are the opposite of each other.

A person may be overly active or not active at all. The depressed may sit in a corner and not say a word, or talk a blue streak even when nobody is listening.

Depressed people are recognized for their tendency to blame themselves for everything. They may declare to the world how worthless and sinful they are. On the other hand, they may also regard themselves as blameless, the victims of others' mishandling and crimes. Paranoid ideas are a common symptom in depression.

The health of depressed people tends to be poor. They often have no appetite and cannot sleep, which affects all the body functions. On the other hand, some may become "health nuts," making a fetish of the right foods and jogging and playing tennis until they drop.

It is also a well-known fact that many depressed people overeat. Obesity is often connected with depression. The tendencies to sleep inordinately long periods and to have difficulty getting up in the morning are also considered symptomatic of depression.

Many depressed persons claim they have no interest in sex. But there are also depressions which have bizarre sexual symptoms. Depressed people tend to be inhibited and repressed in their behavior, yet they are also known to be uncontrolled and impulsive. Suicide is an impulsive act in many cases.

The connecting link in all these symptoms is mood—it is always down, low-key. Even when the defenses are escapist and action-oriented, the unpleasant mood persists.

Sorrow and other strong negative feelings, it must be emphasized, are not necessarily related to depression. They reflect grief, loss, disappointment, concern, and other sad responses that are a part of life itself and justified by life events. Where there are strong feelings there cannot be depression.

Depression represents the absorption of all human feelings, just as black is the absorption of all colors. It is probably no accident that black is the color that represents depression. As a depressed patient remarks, "I don't feel particularly sad about anything. I just feel like that character in the comics who walks about with that black cloud over his head."

Some depressed people are not even aware of their dark mood, only of physical lethargy. Their legs and arms feel heavy, it is difficult to move. They seek excuses for staying put, saying "It's too hot out" or "too cold," or "too much trouble to get dressed." They do not feel particularly sad or low.

Perhaps the surest clue to depression is whether the symptoms lead to withdrawal; giving up of responsibilities; cutting off relationships. If they are accompanied by self-absorption and a lack of caring for others—which is also reflected in a lack of care for one's own appearance and surroundings—one can be quite certain of dealing with a depression.

Depression as "Learned Helplessness"

An interesting and provocative new theory of depression has been developed by psychologist Martin Seligman and his followers—that depression is a feeling of helplessness which is learned from certain life experiences. We can unlearn it, they also maintain, and thereby lose the depression.

First, certain conditions are necessary. We first must have learned to expect something, usually in return for something we have done—a pension check, a rewarding smile, a pleasurable result of some kind. Then suddenly for reasons beyond our control, the reward is no longer forthcoming. The government stops the pension; the person whose smile we received has died. The important thing is that the expected result does not occur *for reasons beyond our control.* There is nothing we can do to bring it about. We are helpless in this regard—we learn the feeling of helplessness.

Had we not learned to expect something we would not feel helpless. Depression results, therefore, from the combination of learned expectation and learned helplessness. Laboratory studies also showed that even when the situation was changed so that individuals could once again have control over things, they never even realized it. They never even tried. The feeling of helplessness persisted and they did nothing, remaining depressed.

It gets more complicated in that there are two kinds of helplessness: universal and personal.

An example of *universal helplessness:* A child contracts an incurable disease and the parents do everything they can to save the child's life. Nothing helps, and despite the best modern medicine had to offer, the child dies. Both parents become depressed; years pass before the mother recovers sufficiently to resume a normal life.

Personal helplessness: a young man is most eager to become a lawyer. He passes all his course work but for some reason cannot pass the bar examination. He takes this exam again and again, studies in special bar preparation courses, but still cannot pass. Eventually, he gives up but he is a marked man forever after. He is depressed and tends to feel himself a failure in almost every new situation.

Which is worse? In both universal and personal helplessness, the people involved learn that no matter what they do, how hard they try, they will not get the desired result. But in the case of the depressed parent, the child's death came from an outside force, and any other parent would have been helpless in the same situation. The death need not affect the parent's sense of self-esteem.

While in the case of the student, the cause was internal. He was stupid: despite all the external assists, he could not pass the test. The source of his trouble came from himself alone. Such a feeling of personal helplessness destroys self-esteem.

Loss of self-esteem is at the core of depression, as mentioned earlier; and the more serious the loss, the more difficult it is to cure the depression. But the most important point psychologist Seligman makes is that since helplessness, whether universal or personal, is a *learned* response, it can be *unlearned*—usually through experiences that restore the feeling of control.

It is an interesting theory. Of course, some questions remain. Why, for instance, did the mother of the sick child suffer such a long-lasting depression? Not all students who fail the bar go through life depressed. Why this particular one? How does one go about motivating a depressed person to unlearn feelings of helplessness?

There are many answers to these questions, and they are dealt with in this theory. The important point here is that unlearning helplessness is possible, and it may even be done on your own. A book titled *Control Your Depression*, by Dr. Peter M. Lewinsohn and his associates (published by Prentice-Hall), is a "self-help" book written in a simple, convenient form for the layman, and it can be very effective.

Does Aging Cause Depression?

It depends on whom you're asking. If you ask people between thirty-five and fifty-five, chances are they will say yes, and make a convincing case. "Why shouldn't old people become depressed? Just think of what happens to them: they lose their spouses, their friends, relatives. Their income is less than before while everything costs more. The children are grown and probably have gone away. They are staring death in the face, and before that maybe a nursing home." How can they not be depressed?

If you ask Dr. Lissy Jarvik, an expert on aging and depression, her answer is quite different. "One of the biggest hurdles we have to overcome is the notion that depression is part of normal aging—it just isn't true."

Considering the depression-making facts of life in older age, Dr. Jarvik says, "Why isn't everybody who's older depressed?"

Depression is not a part of aging. But older people are more often exposed to situations that cause depression than younger people. Even so, Dr. Jarvik points out, a surprisingly small percentage of older people become seriously depressed, only about 10 percent. And if their depression isn't misdiagnosed as "senility," they can be cured. It is quite possible that the very fact of survival into older age itself implies a capacity for dealing with depression.

As for the middle-aged people who took such a gloomy view of depression and old age. What will happen to them when they grow old? Will they be able to cope with depression with their negative attitudes?

Negative or not, at least they have been able to recognize some of the important issues. Now, all they have to do is identify with them—project themselves into the situations they have correctly identified as depression-making and do something about them in advance.

What can be done? Well they can separate facts from fiction, and thus remove some of their own fears. They can (and should) live out—either in the imagination or, better still, in discussions with others—some of the life-crises that cause depression.

The middle-aged participants of one consciousness-raising group chose to act out various situations that they recognized as lying ahead: widowhood, illness, retirement, death, along with some less serious but also depression-making situations, such as getting dentures or face-lifts or going to "fat-farms." They exchanged roles, shifted points of view, and experienced in play-acting various dimensions of each situation.

Did it depress them? Not at all. They came out relieved: it wasn't as bad as they thought, and they were able to get a handle on it. What one couldn't deal with somebody else could. It was a good experience.

Does Fear of Death Cause Depression?

An older person will probably say, "No, I'm not afraid of dying. I just don't want to end up helpless and out of my senses. I especially do not want to be a burden to anyone. Death isn't the problem, it's becoming useless that is."

Ask a younger person about fear of death and you might draw a blank. Although today with books being written about death, "death-therapy" groups, and a cult on death forming, the young person might have gotten into the swing of things and answer, "No, I'm not afraid." But chances are that they are, nevertheless.

Death anxiety is really a younger person's "disease." And while it may appear as a factor in depression, it is really a symptom of the neurotic personality. It is even a major cause of the neurotic's constricted lifestyle. Fear of death prevents the neurotic person from living. However, neurotics actually may have an easier time adjusting to the restrictions society imposes on the elderly because they're used to restrictions and so may make out better than their healthier counterparts!

When death anxiety is a factor in older people's depression, it is usually because of anger that life has short-changed them. Not because they are afraid of dying.

Studies show that people who lead physically active lives and have stimulating social experiences are more accepting of death than those who sleep more and have fewer friends. Death anxiety is not even specifically related to the state of one's health. In fact some studies show a negative relationship between the degree of illness and death anxiety. The human being has ways of dealing even with impending death that prevent anxiety.

The studies agree that aging and illness (the more obvious forerunners of death) do not seem to cause death anxiety. Rather, they indicate that death anxiety is associated with anxiety and maladjustment in general. And perhaps more with youth than with age.

For young people, studies indicate, aging and death are tied together in one unattractive package. Negative attitudes towards the elderly stem from this association of aging with death, and the natural tendency is for young people to experience death anxiety in connection with thoughts of aging and exposure to older people.

How to combat this natural tendency? Again, knowledge and education about aging come to the rescue. Studies prove that when young people are encouraged to talk about death and aging, when they are apprised of the facts, their attitudes improve—both towards old people and their own aging. And those with the highest degree of death anxiety often make the best students!

The Right to Die

Suicide has been given the new name, "Self-Deliverance," by certain groups of aging people. A society of older people called "Hemlock," undoubtedly inspired by Socrates who took his life by drinking poison extracted from the hemlock, pleads their cause with firmness and dignity. They are receiving wide and respectful interest.

To be sure, suicide in old age is a problem—23 percent of suicides committed in the United States are by people over the age of sixty. What's more, most suicide attempts in older age succeed.

More men commit suicide than women even though depression is more common among women in this age group. Possibly, the impact of retirement along with the physical, economic, and emotional losses that occur in older age are more devastating to the self-esteem of men, or the changes in life roles may be sharper and more sudden for men.

Female suicidal behavior is most often related to romantic or marital problems and tends to occur more at earlier ages. Men, it seems, can hold out longer but then may find the fall from status intolerable, as reflected in their higher rate of suicide in later life.

However, with the growing movement toward awareness of self and especially with the more flexible, changing sex roles of recent times, there has been what is called a "spectacular drop" in suicide for the sixty-five- to seventy-four-year-age group. The rate is now less than sixty percent of the 1947 incidence. The social climate is generally more favorable for older people, and life remains inviting to large numbers of people who would not have thought so a couple of generations back.

The openness and spontaneity that is encouraged these days also permits confiding in others, talking over doubts and fears without feelings of constraint. In the past, older people suffered the lack of a confidant, particularly as friends and relatives died off. In modern adult communities people share their problems as well as their pleasures.

Older people, too, retain their sense of independence more easily today; and even though the longer one lives the more crises there are, the traumas are not as great when you can make your own decisions.

The members of Hemlock are not concerned with depression, but with dignity and self-determination at the end of life, as they no doubt were during the course of their lives. If a choice must be made between life and the quality of life, they feel the choice should be their own.

"Psyching" Yourself Out of Trouble

Depression can be prevented in simple, ordinary ways. In fact, "self-monitoring" is probably the only way depression can be prevented, since the individual concerned is the first person to know about it.

But the early, subtle signs of depression, which we usually attribute to something else, may not be recognized and need to be learned.

One early sign is the tendency to stop doing those little daily chores that normally require a push anyway. Not the essentials, like doing the marketing or going to work—that may come later when depression is well on the way—but morning exercises, "duty" phone calls, thank-you notes, and so on.

If this goes on for more than two or three days, it's time to check your mood. How is your mood? Don't ask about "sad" or "happy," but about "heavy," "tired," "bored" or just plain "ugh." Remember, depression creeps up. By the time you know it's there, it can be pretty full-blown.

You don't have to analyze why at this point. There probably isn't any new reason anyway: you'd know if there were. Now is the time to simply *activate* yourself out of it.

Depression cannot coexist with constructive action, so one of the first things to do is force yourself to do at least one of those chores you were avoiding, with the promise of a reward. Give yourself some little present for doing it. And don't worry, it won't lead to gluttony.

After you've passed that first hurdle, you might want to settle back briefly and take stock of yourself. Not of your whole life—there's not much you can do about the past anyway—but of your present life. Are you doing enough with other people?

Never mind that you're self-sufficient or that you've "always been a loner" and enjoyed your own company.

Of course you did: that is why you survived to older age and probably will live a great many years longer. You have lots of inner resources that ought to be used—in the company of other people.

Older people need other people. They need the presence of others to stir up the brain chemistry that prevents depression. There is no need to establish relationships with people you don't like. Just being exposed to them is enough.

Okay, you'll sign up for some courses and go to the weekly meetings. Now, how about some hobbies? Always too busy to develop any? No problem: now is the time.

That will mean work, of course. New interests do not come naturally, and there will have to be some input on your part without immediate returns. But trust the old libido, and soon forced interest turns into genuine pleasure, real "gutsy" satisfaction. One thing will lead to another, and you will not let yourself be depressed again!

But Something More May Be Needed

Let's say your score on the depression questionnaire showed mild to moderate depression. If only you could manage those few seemingly simple steps we just outlined, how wonderful it would be—but your problem is motivation. You cannot get going.

But you're not ready to see a shrink, you want to handle this yourself. You could try a little free association along the lines mentioned in the chapter on memory loss. But we'll add a few more steps.

First some "relaxation therapy." Lie down where it is quiet and you won't be disturbed. Now breathe slowly, not necessarily deeply (that will come naturally), but from your stomach, not your chest. As it happens, you'll feel yourself relaxing.

Now tighten your toes and relax them. Tighten your whole foot and relax it; then your other foot. Tighten every part of you, and then relax it, proceeding right up to your scalp. This is to make you aware of the feeling of tension and relaxation so that in case you tense up somewhere as you are lying there (a signal that something is going on with your emotions), you'll be able to relax it.

Now you're ready to clear your mind and let whatever thoughts are waiting outside to come in. You'll watch for those that cause tension (just as you did for memory loss) and either free-associate or deal with them directly as they come up.

Anger is the main emotion in depression—anger that is unresolved and that cannot be directed where it belongs. Some even believe that people who kill themselves really want to kill someone else. A very important therapy called "antidepressive therapy" works by enraging patients almost to violence, at which point everyone surrounds the patient and urges yelling, weeping, or whatever brings relief—except hurting oneself or others. It usually works.

But all you will have to do is simply identify your feelings of anger, and the object of it. In your state of relaxation you will see things in a clearer perspective, without anxiety. You may come up with some solutions, or just decide it is something that will have to be tolerated. You may decide to pursue it further with a professional. In any case you won't waste time or energy on depression.

But you're only human, and every now and then you'll get a pang or two. That is when to apply *stop therapy*. It's a bona fide therapy that consists of your shouting "Stop!" to yourself, aloud or in your head, whenever an anger-making or depressive thought starts the pangs going. Cleared of the pangs, you can go about your business. But don't forget to deal with the problem-thoughts later when you relax.

But It Isn't Me—It's My Husband

Nothing makes the "well" one feels more frustrated and helpless than having to watch a mate or a parent sink into a depression. First of all the early symptoms are so grating—irritability, uncooperativeness, even uncleanliness. And it takes a while to realize that he or she may actually be digging away at you, purposely, to make you angry.

The stubbornness, the silences, the bursts of temper—these don't seem like depression—but more like hatred. They are: self-hatred.

In older age, the symptoms of depression, like the symptoms of "senility," seem to appear with a suddenness and severity that makes extreme measures often necessary. By the time the depression is recognized it may be full-blown and unmanageable at home. The earlier signs are usually attributed to "getting older."

Obviously, it is too late to "psyche" oneself out of this depression. Professional help is needed. But the family is still essential: First, to stand guard against professionals who may stereotype the problem as "senility"; and second, to keep the "welcome mat" out so that the depressed one knows there is an end to the journey into sickness and that end is back at home again. This makes recovery possible. Otherwise there may be no reason to forfeit the depression.

There are many approaches to depression in older people that are bringing good results, including drugs and psychotherapy. New studies of thyroid and other hormone functions are opening up other pathways of treatment.

Depression is one of the curable diseases of aging. But of course, early detection and prevention are preferred.

How to Beat Depression in Later Life

In some ways it's easier than in earlier life. Because people who live longer have learned the habits of good mental and physical hygiene that conquer depression.

In some ways though, it's harder because there are more causes for depression in older age.

What to do? I hope you've gotten some good ideas here. The rest is better said by Dr. V.E. Frankl in *The Doctor and the Soul:* "Meaning is unique and specific to each man alone. . . Death is actually a factor in life's meaningfulness. . . The issue is not that life has no meaning. . . but that if death has no meaning, life has none either."

Where there is fear of death, there can be no purpose in life.

Chapter Seven

The Big Three of Aging

Food—Friends—Exercise

"It takes all the running you can do to keep in the same place."
Red Queen in *Alice in Wonderland*

Preserve What You've Got

That's the secret of successful aging.

You eat to *keep* fit. You exercise to *keep* muscle. You socialize to *keep* friends, or more important, to *keep* the habit of contact.

The big difference between young and old is the *replacement factor*. It takes longer to put back in what you take out, except for weight, of course.

Good nutrition, good muscle tone, and a piece of the action—these are the three most important elements in the good life. Ask any centenarian.

In fact, a great many centenarians have been asked in recent years as to what they attributed their longevity. The answer is invariably: careful diet, regular exercise, and continued involvement in community affairs.

127

Even in unpolluted regions of the world where nature holds sway and people live long, the ones who live the longest abide by these three rules.

Eat Less—Live Longer

Many years ago the noted geriatrician, J.T. Freeman claimed that a key mechanism in retarding aging is the reduction of food intake. He also noted that reduced food intake retards both the onset and progression of chronic disease.

Since that time, many studies in the lab and outside have proven that low-calorie diets (in animal studies, these can even be near-starvation diets) prolong life. There's a catch to it, however. While one may live longer on the lesser food intake, one also becomes weaker. So some adjustments must be made to combine lesser calories with high nutrition.

How many calories should one consume daily? The following chart gives the recommended average allowances for men and women starting at age sixty.

Age	Women	Men
60–64	1730	2400
65–69	1680	2350
70–74	1630	2280
75–79	1580	2210
80–84	1510	2110
85–89	1440	2020
90+	1400	2000

These figures coincide with the calories in the diets of those well-publicized, long-lived citizens of Abkhazia in Russia and also those who live along the Syrian border in Turkey. Although reports of their life spans are probably exaggerated (upwards of 130 years in some cases), they are undoubtedly enjoying very long lives and remain remarkably active throughout.

Their diets, of course, are simple and free of "additives." They eat plenty of fresh fruits and vegetables. Grapes, persimmons, pomegranates, and nuts (which may be a factor in keeping them clear of cholesterol) are eaten freely. Some meat is eaten, simply prepared and usually broiled. And sugar has been replaced by honey. It is claimed that the ones who live to be 100 have never had a toothache.

Buttermilk is a favorite drink; yogurt is a staple. But water is taboo. Wine is drunk instead, at breakfast, dinner, and supper—and may be help in destroying microbes in the large amounts of uncooked food which are eaten. But no coffee or tea! In addition to all the wine, it is the custom to drink two shots of vodka—twice a day.

These diets may not be applicable to us—or even be responsible for their longevity, but one thing is certain. The 2000-calories daily intake seems related to longevity, and we can certainly plan around that.

At first glance, 2000 calories may not seem like a great deal of food. But it represents a handsome amount of good eating—even gourmet dining—if you go easy on the desserts, liquor, and "empty" calories in general.

There are many books available on diet, so we will not go into specifics here, just some general principles.

First, by reducing the actual volume of food eaten you will aid the digestive process. Many problems of digestion, and absorption of nutrients, can be avoided by following the principle of eating smaller portions at one time and allowing more time for digestion. Even people with gall bladder and liver problems will find this helpful.

Second, avoid starches and sugar as much as possible. They are not as easily metabolized as you grow older. In addition they add weight without adding a commensurate amount of energy.

Focus on the proteins, along with a small amount of fat, and go heavy on foods that are rich in vitamins, particularly B and C (the green leafy vegetables). Be sure to get your calcium.

Obviously, each individual has different needs and tolerances for the various foods essential to maintaining health. There are aids to digestion—i.e., for milk and certain raw vegetables—that can be used. Food supplements such as vitamins, iron, and other minerals are also most helpful but should be taken under medical guidance.

Big Returns for a Small Investment

The smaller amount of food you eat as you grow older can have powerful results, just where you want them. A small packet of unflavored gelatins for instance, taken daily in fruit juice or vegetable juices will thicken your hair, strengthen your nails, and give your skin resilience. And it amounts to only a few calories—an excellent mid-morning snack that will also control your hunger and let you eat less at lunch.

Calcium from milk, cheese, and meat (eaten judiciously of course with cholesterol in mind) is not only good for the bones but will stop foot cramps as well.

The point is you can eat to help correct problems that are specific to aging. It is well worth a little research on your part to explore the possibilities of lecithin, vitamin E, niacin, thiamin, and folacin. Your local health food dealer will have lots of information to help you out. In this age of "pill-popping," many medications rob us of the nutrients that are in our foods, and there are things we can, and should do about that, too.

Many signs of "aging" such as irritability, moodiness, depression, and even "senility" are due to malnutrition and are corrected by eating the proper foods. According to Dr. Arnold Schaefer, head of the

University of Nebraska Nutrition Center, even certain brain disorders are cleared in a few hours after eating an egg omelet.

Exercise for Brain Power

Up to about age twenty five you exercise to improve your physique, enhance your appearance, increase your strength and endurance. After that you exercise to keep it all that way.

And after fifty you exercise to keep one more thing in good shape—your mind. Yes, the same routines that broadened your shoulders and flattened your stomach will keep the brain cells growing right through life.

Consider the "miracles" that resulted from an exercise program, run by Dr. Herbert A. DeVries, of the University of Southern California Gerontology Center. Not only did the group of older men who participated in his exercise program function better physically and mentally, but a vigorous fifteen-minute walk reduced tension more effectively than 400 milligrams of a tranquilizer. Men with a life history of migraine headaches found their headaches gone after a few weeks of physical training.

A group of "high-fit" men, ages twenty four to sixty eight, were compared with a group of "low-fit" men of the same ages after a program of physical fitness exercises (jogging, calisthenics, running, and self-selected sports). Regardless of age, the high-fit group had a significantly higher intelligence score than the low-fit, on the before-and-after tests.

Not only was more oxygen circulated to the brain because of the exercise, but along with it came more glucose which is the essential nutrient of the brain. Exercise, according to this study, actually *reverses* the destructive biochemical and physiological changes that are believed to occur in aging.

Beware of Muscle Hunger

It happens often in the civilized world and starts in childhood—with busing to school, long hours in front of TV, the rage for "brain-games" instead of ballgames. We starve our muscles.

Muscles feed on exercise. Being quiet starves them, breaking down the physiological control system of the body, and directly weakens the heart.

Russian scientists believe that it is not the strain, worry, and rapid pace of modern life that harms us, but the relaxed living and lack of exercise. Exercise builds up body proteins even if you cannot eat sirloin steak. It is necessary to put into your bones the calcium you get in your diet. Even with the best of diets, rest and relaxation rob the bones of calcium.

Osteoporosis, or softening of the bones, has always been considered a female disease of aging because so many more older women came down with it. However, it may well be that lack of exercise is a strong factor in bringing about this disease in women. It will be interesting to see whether it will decrease as women become more and more athletic.

Russian specialists say that muscle hunger is a major cause of heart disease and believe in preventive exercise. Naturally, an exercise program should be started at an easy pace and the load gradually increased. It seems the more you feed your muscles with exercise, the more they want—which is why you find yourself needing more laps in the pool, longer walks, or heavier barbells to get a feeling of satisfaction.

Even quite old people will grow stronger and stronger and need increasing amounts of exercise. The main factor working against them is their *psychological inhibitions*. In a study of men in their seventies, they consciously and unconsciously prevented themselves from exerting the effort they were actually capable of.

When they became less cautious, their gain in strength was equal to that of younger people, a finding that was somewhat surprising to both the investigators and subjects.

Posture to Prevent Aging

... and prolong life. "The diseases of old age are postural," Dr. J. T. Freeman has said. He traces many of the diseases of old age to postural changes due to the pull of gravity, which causes collapse of the body column and misalignment of muscles and limbs.

Not only are various organs affected—kidney, intestines, and heart to name a few—but bones, tissue, circulation, blood pressure, and body chemistry are also impaired by postural changes. A major change is in the pelvic area, which becomes compressed vertically and expanded laterally.

Are these changes inevitable along with the diseases they cause? Dr. Freeman points out that, "Animals have shapes and forms. Only man has posture. . ."

We can do something about posture. Exercise in older age should be geared to maintain good posture. This means strengthening the back and upper torso, the diaphragm and the arms. The legs usually get sufficient exertion, and since they are also closer to the ground, they do not get the same pull of gravity as the upper parts of the body.

A good principle to remember in maintaining posture through exercise is to focus on undoing the pull of gravity. The best are stretching exercises or yoga-type exercises, which are geared to reverse the pull of gravity.

And while we're on the subject of yoga, scientists have come up with an interesting new twist on breathing which seems to contradict the ancient laws. It seems deep breathing is not necessary, at least, not while exercising. In fact, it might be harmful: the extra carbon dioxide which is produced by exercise is necessary for the proper feeding of the muscles. They really do not need the increased oxygen from deep breathing. It's the carbon dioxide which improves circulation, and the more physically-fit you become the less the need for deep breathing. According to the theory.

Activity as a Life Style

Ideally, there should be no need for exercise as a special activity. In countries where there is unusual longevity, there are few golf courses and tennis courts and people have not heard of calisthenics. Life is exercise. And while there may be no direct proof that their active lives are responsible for their longevity, there is proof that inactivity leads to early death.

In the Duke University longevity studies, it was found that people who had difficulty walking lived to only about 80 percent of their projected lifespan. People who were in wheelchairs, or bed-bound, lived to only about 64 percent.

On the other hand, those whose mobility was unimpaired lived far beyond expectancy, in fact half again as long as they were expected to!

The active life has its problems, of course. Arthritis can hit tender points, no matter what the lifestyle and no matter what one may call it—"tennis elbow," "jogger's knee" or "sheep-tender's wrist."

There is even an arthritic "personality type" which in a way is the kind our society admires. Arthritic personalities tends to be perfectionistic, demanding of themselves, and effective in their chosen area of activity. They dislike the effects of tranquilizers and use drugs and alcohol sparingly. They also relax poorly.

But even in arthritis, exercise is the cure for what it actually may have caused—corrective exercise, that is, which restores balance between unequally used parts of the body. In fact, as you get older you should exercise to balance strength so that stress points cannot develop. Many health clinics focus on individual imbalances and prescribe exercises to bring them into proper body alignment.

Exercise Keeps You Young

It really does. And not only in the way you look and feel, although most of us would be glad to settle for that. But also under the microscope. Skin, tissue, organs and bones all display the components of youth, and are even indistinguishable from youth in the person who stays physically fit.

The time-honored stereotype that you "slow down" as you get older is not true—in the physically active person.

Recent studies show that the "slow-down" is due to lack of physical fitness and not to age. Athletes have faster reaction times than nonathletes no matter what their ages. When older people do slow down, it is only at the *decision point* of a particular movement, while their rate of speed itself is generally unaffected.

These studies prove the best protection against slowing down is physical activity which, unlike mental activity, stimulates metabolism, respiration, blood circulation, digestion, and the glands and keeps you alert.

Exercise keeps you young because it maintains your body's rhythm of compensation and adaptation. By pacing yourself and balancing the forces of your particular lifestyle, you help prevent the patches of deterioration which signal old age. With good body rhythm, there is less untimely wearing out of particular organs or functions. Changes are gradual, not blatantly noticeable.

You look young because you *are* young—biologically.

Avoid Social Aging

Okay, you know how to avoid psychological and biological aging, but that's not where it ends. There's a third kind of aging: social aging.

This means being put on the shelf by society. It also means putting yourself on the shelf because it's not worth the fight.

It *is* worth the fight. Because, society's attitudes lag behind society's realities. Take retirement: we're still following outmoded laws and conditions that no longer exist. The talents of older people are needed, often desperately so, and their skills are marketable. This is being proven all over the country, but it requires constant effort to beat down the hold of the stereotypes.

Society's role in bringing about social aging is fairly apparent. Of more concern here is the role of individuals in aiding and abetting their own social aging.

Disengagement theory is no more than an observation of how older people bring about their own social aging. They don't start the process, society does that. But they carry it through.

How Insecure Are You?

Here are common things that make some people feel tense or fearful. Check off the ones that apply to you. If you've checked off more than five, you're pretty uptight—can't be having much fun.

- ☐ loud voices
- ☐ speaking in public
- ☐ failing at something
- ☐ being teased
- ☐ meeting strangers
- ☐ people in authority
- ☐ tough-looking, noisy, young people
- ☐ being watched while you're working
- ☐ criticism

- ☐ angry people
- ☐ being ignored
- ☐ looking foolish
- ☐ making mistakes
- ☐ making small talk
- ☐ forgetting names

Nature's Shrinking Man—Or Woman

Even in the normal course of aging, people become more vulnerable and defensive. They shrink from society. On the Rorschach Test (the inkblot test), aging people who seem to be making it pretty well on the outside reveal their inner feelings of insecurity and inferiority. These feelings are not conscious, but they influence behavior in subtle ways.

An example is the man who proclaims his retirement status too loudly. His car's license plate reads: "LAZY RP," RP standing for "retired person." Another is people who exhaust themselves in leisure-time activities—not for pleasure but to quell their resentment, which invariably bursts forth inappropriately and with disastrous social results.

This kind of social contact is not likely to promote happiness, although it is better than no contact. But the underlying problem is that because of society's old-fashioned attitudes, many older people eventually do give up their contacts. Or put another way, they give up the fight. They avoid challenging situations and force themselves to take a backseat. They agree that younger is better in business and government. They accept the stereotypes.

But do they really mean it? Here is a list of current one-liners, and you can judge for yourself.

How I Know I'm Growing Older
- Everything hurts, and what doesn't hurt doesn't work.

- The gleam in my eyes is from the sun hitting my bifocals.
- I feel like the night before, and I haven't been anywhere.
- My little black book contains only names ending in M.D.
- I get winded playing chess.
- My children begin to look middle-aged.
- I finally reached the top of the ladder and found it leaning against the wrong wall.
- I join a health club and don't go.
- I begin to outlive enthusiasm.
- I decide to procrastinate but then never get around to it.
- I'm still chasing women, but can't remember why.
- My mind makes contracts my body can't meet.
- A dripping faucet causes an uncontrollable bladder urge.
- I know all the answers, but nobody asked me the questions.
- I look forward to a dull evening.
- I walk with my head held high trying to get used to my bifocals.
- My favorite part of my newspaper is "25 Years Ago Today."
- I turn out the lights for economic rather than romantic reasons.
- I sit in a rocking chair and can't get it going.
- My knees buckle and my belt won't.
- I regret resisting temptation.
- I'm 17 around the neck, 42 around the waist, and 96 around the golf course.
- I stop looking forward to my next birthday.
- After painting the town red, I have to take a long rest before applying a second coat.
- Dialing a long-distance call wears me out.
- I'm startled the first time I'm addressed as "old-timer."

- I remember today that yesterday was our wedding anniversary.
- I just can't stand people who are intolerant.
- The best part of the day is over when the alarm clock goes off.
- I burn the midnight oil at 9 p.m.
- My back goes out more than I do.
- A fortune-teller offers to read my face.
- My pacemaker makes the garage door go up when I watch a pretty girl go by.
- I get my exercise acting as pallbearer for my friends who exercise.
- I have too much room in the house and not enough in the medicine cabinet.
- I sink my teeth into a steak and they stay there.
- It takes me all night to do what I used to do all night.

Saved—By a Sense of Humor

Well, if you can laugh at these jokes things can't be all that bad.

In fact laughter can cure you when the doctors give up on you, as the famous case of Norman Cousins has proven. Stricken by a "hopeless" disease, he prescribed his own medicine, laughter; and it worked. We have a great deal to learn from his book, *Anatomy of an Illness*.

A sense of humor—and a sense of future. Plan activities with others and plan them ahead. A group of older people were evaluated by various ratings as to their health, happiness, and feelings of usefulness. The results showed that all of these good things were associated with having future activities. All the high scorers on the ratings kept date books and had future commitments.

Many other studies have shown the value of keeping a fix on the future as a means of maintaining mental health. It figures, of course. People who look forward must have a sound sense of themselves, and of their place in society.

How did they get this sound sense of themselves? By remaining socially active, by having enough good times to cancel out the bad times. By having new experiences in order to learn to correct past mistakes.

Those one-liners poked fun at old age. But the people who can laugh at them can take growing older in stride—along with everything else.

Social Ties for Longer Life

At a recent symposium the topic was the importance of social ties for maintaining health and prolonging life. And this is not only because social activity is so stimulating to mind and body.

It seems that people who are socially involved also take protective and preventive health measures so that they can remain socially involved. They want to look and feel good and be acceptable to others—and they are willing to work at it.

Their social relationships in turn provide them with help in coping with their problems. In small towns where everybody knows each other, the crises of retirement and widowhood are much less drastic than they are in urban areas where isolation is the rule.

In one study of men who lost their jobs after a plant closed down, the men who had strong social ties adjusted much more easily and got themselves new jobs.

Social ties are not to be confused with social supports. They are almost opposites. Social supports means "help is on the way." Social ties means "help me to help myself." Social ties involves mutual give-and-take, but the responsibility, the decision-making, the control always rest with each individual.

People with social ties have more resistance to illness. It was once thought that poor people had more illness because of their poverty. Now it is thought that it might be due to their social marginality. Japanese men who were relocated in areas where they had no social ties suffered more heart attacks than a comparison group living in their normal setting.

Everybody needs somebody, even if it's only a pet. Another study showed that patients live longer after a heart attack when they have a pet for company! Or a plant. Nursing home patients who are given a plant to take care of live longer than those who have nothing to care for.

States that are comprised of smaller communities and few large cities report less stress-related illness. While this is not surprising, Dr. J. T. Freeman suggests that a certain amount of stress is good for you as you grow older. It may prevent deterioration and even aid survival by arousing and mobilizing the body's resources.

Many older people survive where younger ones succumb because of their experience in handling stress. Certainly, this has been corroborated in recent studies of survivorship after floods and other catastrophies where older people did very well.

However, "stress" is not to be confused with "strain" which can deplete the body's reserves.

Want to Live to Be 100?

Lots of people are living that long, and longer. And not just in Russia, Turkey, and Ecuador, where citizens have been making the headlines as they sail well past the century mark.

Right here in the United States, according to the 1980 census there are 32,000 Americans over the age of 100. True, they may be a bit feeble at this point, but they did fine in their eighties and nineties, judging from the comparatively small percentage in nursing homes.

In any case, these centenarians are not complaining. "My mother lived to be 100," said a 125-year-old man, "and my father—140. Why should I live less? Let us drink to your health and not worry about mine."

In Abkhazia, Russia, labor is believed to be a major cause of longevity. The Abkhazian views work as life itself. A group of people all over 100 continued working on a collective farm even though they received pensions which were sufficient to satisfy all their needs. Work is essential to the normal activity of all body organs. To stop work would mean to stop the body's rhythm established over so many decades.

What kind of work do they do? What they always did: chopping firewood, digging in gardens, mowing and gathering the hay. Many choose not to go on pension, and a person who has reached pension age cannot be dismissed because of his age. One shepherd of 120 years experience insisted on continuing work even though he was 139 years old. There is a philosophy that a person cannot "live too long" in Abkhazia. Old people are respected and important in the community, and they claim never to experience melancholy or loneliness.

Of course, they stick to 2000 calories a day, and consider "fat" to be synonymous with "sick."

Asked whether a fountain of youth existed in Abkhazia, a 138-year-old woman replied, "Of course it exists . . . it is inside each of us. Only not everyone knows how to use it."

People in more "civilized" areas shudder at the thought of living to be 100, because they assume it means sickness, helplessness, and deterioriation. Not so. People live so long because they are healthy; longevity implies good health. In one study of the long-lived in Turkey, almost all (94 percent) still had their vision and could hear adequately. Only 24 percent had a partial hearing defect. Only 14 percent were housebound.

But all the subjects in this study were mentally competent and able to interact with others. In Turkey, interestingly, two thirds of those who live to the 100 mark are men, and they are men of medium height for the most part. "Don't be too tall or you'll get caught," say the Turks. "Don't be too short or you'll get squashed." And practically none of them smoke.

How to Reach 100 in the USA

So far it seems to be continued employment, education, physical fitness, inner contentment, and no smoking which contribute to long life.

The higher the education the better the chances for a long life. Professors live longer than farmers who have less than a high school education. Professors seem to have a better life expectancy than almost anyone, and there's probably a lesson to be learned in that.

Certain types of employment are clearly safer than others. Perhaps professors live longer not only because their work is satisfying and respect-commanding, but also because they usually walk across campus to work and don't have to battle subways and freeways.

Higher-status occupations not only provide safer and healthier working conditions but also more income for health care, nutrition, and housing. Although physical health by itself is the most important predictor of longevity, when education and type of occupation are added together they make a more important indicator than health.

In this country as elsewhere, continued employment is a factor in promoting longevity, along with exercise, social stimulation, and sensible diet.

One expected factor did not show up in a recent study: married people did not live longer than the widowed or divorced. Actually, single people seemed to have a slight edge. The opposite was generally true in the past. Married people did live longer. However, recent studies are beginning to associate longevity with the single state. Perhaps it is due to our changing times.

It is interesting that the reports do not seem to be concerned with heredity as a factor in longevity, except to note that one's potential lifespan and actual lifespan are usually very different. A person who has inherited the expectation of a very long lifespan may be outlived by someone who has not. The investigations of Russian longevity point out the multinational ancestry of the long-lived and claim it was the mixture of genes that contributed to longevity, not the inheritance of just one line of genes.

Longevity is not a mere accident of birth. There are good reasons why people live long lives: good work, good health, good nature—all contribute to longevity.

How Inevitable Is Old Age?

Many of the inevitable changes of old age, Dr. Lissy Jarvik thinks, may really be chance occurrences. And that include wrinkles, loss of hair, thinning of the bones, and vision and hearing losses. She believes these are changes due mainly to ecological conditions and dietary, chemical, and hormonal factors, and not necessarily to underlying biological change.

They come about, Dr. Jarvik maintains, because of the things we do—not because of age—and as such, they can be prevented. However, the expectation that they are inevitable prevents us from doing something about these changes in advance. For example: reading with proper lighting, staying out of the sun, and taking in sufficient vitamins and hormones.

Dr. Jarvik's most interesting and encouraging point of view is that even genetic traits are not necessarily inevitable but are alterable. And so, the laws of aging may not be immutable.

Chapter Eight

Swinging After Sixty

"So long as men can breathe, or eyes can see
So long lives [love], and this gives life to
thee."

Shakespeare

Sex in Older People

Is there sex after sixty? After seventy? Later? Do older
people really want sex, or do they think they *should*
want it?

Sex is a possibility throughout life, most investigators agree. Though, not everyone over sixty
wants sex, or can have it if they do. As with younger
people, sex is part of a relationship, and for some people,
sex cannot exist without a relationship. For others, the
relationship they have prevents sex.

Young people usually cannot accept the fact of sex
in older people. In hospitals, the old patient who makes a
pass at the young nurse is not only the butt of many
popular jokes, but also considered a very real problem in
nurses' training.

But, he is just doing what comes naturally, only he forgot that young women are turned off by old men who make passes. (They don't react that way when young patients make passes.) Young nurses should be trained to intercept these passes without making the patient feel he's less a man because he is old.

Recently, some rather startling scientific facts proved that the sex drive per se goes on and on. In one study, men in their sixties had night erections while they were dreaming during 22 percent of their total sleep time. They averaged over three sexy episodes per night, each one lasting an average of almost 24 minutes; and some men had as many as six such episodes a night.

In another study, men ranging in age from seventy-one to ninety-six (with an average age of about eighty) had erections during 75 percent of their dream periods. As a matter of fact, they were "sexier" than a group of sixty- to sixty-nine-year-olds in the same study who had erections during only 64 percent of their dream periods.

True, men in their twenties and thirties have higher rates of erection during their dreams, but why quibble about a few percentage points when older citizens make such a respectable showing? Older men, by the way, have almost twice as much penile action as younger men when there is no dreaming during sleep, a puzzling fact since we have been led to believe that the older we get the more erotic stimulation we need.

Women, of course, have been coming away with the honors in terms of sexual response for some time now. All studies corroborate that women retain the capacity for orgasm right through life. But have they been taking advantage of this unusual talent? Far from it! Women who are upwards of sixty today, we are told, were immobilized by guilt, fear, inhibition, and shame in their earlier years. When release finally comes after menopause, male partners are either "incapable," reluctant, or deceased.

A lack of partners notwithstanding, even women who never attained orgasm in their younger years often have sex dreams complete with orgasm during and after menopause. Masturbation, sex researcher Alfred Kinsey found, is a more appropriate index of female sexuality than any other, and it declines only slightly, if at all with aging.

Masturbation, it appears, is an important sexual outlet for all older people, men and women, married and unmarried alike. A study of married men ranging in age from sixty-five to ninety-two who continued to have sex with their wives from one to four times a month also engaged in masturbation in about 25 percent of the cases.

The shortage and staleness of partners so often given as reasons for the slackening of sex after age sixty may have to be reevaluated. The question might well be asked: Are partners necessary? For sexual release, that is. Of course they are necessary for a relationship, which may be more important than sex in the long run.

So now the question becomes, is sex necessary? It is, otherwise why would it go on and on, with both men and women, even if only in their dreams?

Sex and the Stale Marriage

In long-lasting marriages, it is usually the man who draws the line on sex, and he does it at just the time when his wife, finally rid of those earlier inhibitions, is rarin' to go. (Researchers say that women do not reach their peak of sexual drive until middleage.)

Obviously, if women do not swing after sixty (and most of them do not), it is not because of a waning sex drive. So why with all that female potential do men tend to turn away from sex, except when they are safely asleep and dreaming? The stale marriage syndrome—

familiarity, boredom, resentment, and regret—is probably a major cause of the removal of sex from the marriage bed.

Where does it go? One place it goes is to the health spa. There is something very sexy about a spa, and many older men, and some women may even prefer it to the real thing. It's easy, there's no hassle, and you don't have to prove a thing. You just lie there and let the patting, stroking, kneading and steaming, the hot towels, cold towels, and Jacuzzi do all the work. If you feel like working at it, you can do the "Sexercises" which stress the pelvis as the pivotal point. And who could object to that? Especially since it is the best way to narrow the broadening of the beam which takes place during aging.

Spas are respectable. The best golf clubs have them, and mature people, even those in their seventies and eighties go there. Spas are fun; they serve a good purpose, too. They let you relax without guilt and be sensual without shame. Bodies look better in the spa because they feel so good (and, in any case, the others are not so great either). Spas can get a stale-marriage spouse out of the house and off the hook. By sublimating the sex drive in this way, spas insure keeping it alive and well until the right moment and keep you feeling good all over while you're waiting.

Something Else Is Needed

Neither spas nor sex promote marriage, unfortunately. Despite the growing population of people over sixty five, there has been no increase in marriages among the older. The statistics still show only 3 brides per 1000 single older women and 17 grooms per 1000 single older men.

Marriage opportunities plummet every five years for women. Between sixty five and sixty nine, chances are twice what they are between the ages seventy and seventy-four. The rates for men decline, too, but not so precipitously. As with younger people, the divorced are more likely to remarry than the widowed, and the never-marrieds are least likely to take the plunge in their later years.

Unfortunately as well, neither sex nor spas alone can revive the stale marriage that has a big buildup of resentment and regret. If, over the years a lot of emotional bills have gone unpaid because the spouses have put up and shut up instead of bringing things out in the open and leveling with each other, it may take marital counseling or individual psychotherapy to straighten matters out. And for some, even that may not work. There has been a remarkable increase in divorce among couples over sixty five in recent years.

Any drive, particularly the sex drive, suffers from too much of the same stimulus. A drive develops in intensity according to what the outside world has to offer in terms of excitation and satisfaction. Even long-devoted pairs of laboratory mice, blissful in their individual cages where they live as couples, tend to give up sex after a while, causing all sorts of problems with the experiments. But when one inspired scientist decided to put three pairs of mice in the same cage, the sexual activity in all six aging mice zoomed upward! The same method worked with several aging monkeys when they were provided with new, though not necessarily young mates. Everyone benefited from the change and the experiments could proceed.

In view of all this, it would seem that "swinging after sixty," with all the variation, stimulation, and excitement it implies, would be a very good idea for keeping the sexual fires burning. Why then are there not more people over sixty doing it instead of just dreaming it?

Where Are All the "Dirty Old Men?"

It seems that the "dirty old man" stereotype is exactly that, a stereotype. Sexual crimes comprise the lowest percentage of crimes in those over sixty-five, the number being almost infinitesimal in comparison with younger men. The fact is that sexual deviance in older age is grossly misrepresented and exaggerated and the statistics prove it.

Not that it does not occur. There are instances of elderly men suddenly resorting to child molestation, homosexuality, prostitutes, and other unaccustomed (for them) sexual acts. This does not happen to be true of elderly women, but might perhaps be so if the culture sanctioned sexual license for them, and if opportunity permitted. Or perhaps it has simply been unreported. In recent studies more intensive interviewing techniques have been uncovering sexual deviance in older women as well.

When there is sexual deviance among older people, it is usually not so much representative of sexual drive as it is symptomatic of other, often unrelated psychiatric or physical problems and should be regarded and treated as such. It may be a sign of depression or it may be a danger signal preceding cerebral hemmorhage. It may follow an incapacitating illness or emotional loss. It may be a last-ditch defense against death-panic.

Interestingly, in illnesses actually related to sexual function, such as prostate disorder, bizarre sexual behavior rarely occurs. On the contrary, there is a tendency for sexual activity to decline after prostectomy, although it is not a consistent tendency and occurs mainly among men who do not have partners with whom they feel familiar and comfortable. Most men retain their sexual potency after the operation, and in some cases, potency which was previously lost may be regained.

Sex and Sickness
When there are bizarre sexual symptoms in connection with illness, they are often unrecognized as such. An

elderly man recovering from a stroke complained of severe spasms in the area of his groin, which would cause him to double up in pain, bringing several female attendants to his side. Back in bed after much attention and fussing, his nonparalyzed hand never left the area of his groin, opening and closing and clutching interminably. Never once did the possibility of sexual frustration come up in the rehabilitation conference. Instead, the patient was subjected to every conceivable test and procedure related to muscle spasm.

Needless to say, all results were negative.

It is accepted among experienced physicians who work with older patients that many physical complaints and illnesses reflect indirect sexual drive disturbances, or actually cause it. Among these are cancer, arthritis, kidney failure, back pain, arteriosclerosis, stroke, and almost any terminal illness.

Women, particularly, may develop a variety of problems in the genital, urethral and anal areas without clearly discernible physical causes. On the other hand, there are diseases affecting those areas which are sexually stimulating and lead to sexual frustration in the absence, one could say, of actual sexual drive.

There is an interesting parallel to this situation in the Rorschach testing of older people. The Rorschach or inkblot test is a test of personality in which people are asked to imagine different things they might see in pictures of enlarged inkblots. Certain parts of the inkblots have sexual connotations for most younger people. But older people, although they are obviously attracted to those parts, tend to turn a sex symbol into some other body part. They will see a "kidney" where a younger person might see a "penis," or a "heart" instead of a "vagina." Of course one can interpret this in several different ways, but all point to a displacement of sex to other bodily functions and possibly to illness itself as a source of sexual gratification.

Off-Limits Sex

Bizarre sexual behavior, on the rare occasions when it occurs among the elderly, is usually not due to sex. Over-sixty swingers are the exception rather than the rule. Massage parlors are still regarded as off-limits for respectable men and don't exist for women, even though the variety and stimulation they offer may indeed be the best medicine for the stale-marriage syndrome.

And while pornography, X-rated movies, and sexual "surrogates" are now being dignified as "sex therapy" for the younger population, what clinic would dare recommend them to the seventy-five-year-old immobilized by a stroke, or the grandmother who has suddenly taken to wandering in the streets in her nightgown?

Sometimes, too much sexual freedom can prove downright dangerous for older people. In a recent nursing home study, it turned out that some patients' previous sexual activities had brought about their institutionalization. They had lived with lovers, had homosexual affairs or other sexual alliances which the family had concealed for years. When the victimized spouse died, the children refused responsibility for the offending parent and eventually placed them in the nursing home. There, the culprits gleefully revealed the sensational facts of their lives, unreformed and unremorseful to the end.

Perhaps the best solution to the "dirty old man" problem is more dirty old women. Although there are no official studies yet, there are indications of lively innovations being introduced among the current vigorous and sophisticated generation of over-sixties, ranging from Jacuzzi encounter sessions to the enterprising use of vibrators. Even as this is being written, the problem may be resolving itself.

The Stranger in the Mirror

Most older people will tell you that they really have not changed "inside," and psychological tests prove it again and again. Once older people are relaxed and responding without anxiety, it is almost impossible to tell their ages from a psychological test.

The hardest part for the unchanging "inner man" to accept is the bodily changes which are inevitable with aging.

"Instant senility" may follow a paralyzing stroke, hip fracture, or even a first set of full dentures. Of course, this is not really senility but a crisis breakdown, the crisis being old age and the cause being whatever physical changes represent "the beginning of the end" for a particular individual.

It goes deeper than that, far back into infancy. Body image has nothing to do with sex, although it can cause havoc with a person's sex life. An infant is conscious of its body only in terms of what it does, never in terms of what it looks like. If it works and brings gratification, it is good. If it does not work, if it causes frustration, it is bad. Later on, good and bad become beautiful and ugly, desirable and rejected, trustworthy and dangerous. Of course, people grow to develop more positive ideas about themselves and are not necessarily ruled by those early negative self-feelings. However, when one's defenses are down, for whatever reason, there can be a return to the subjective irrationality of the infant, especially in terms of one's body image.

Disturbances in body image are a crucial trap for the older person who is already hard-pressed to meet the continuing crises which come with normal aging. The body that does not perform the way it used to may be psychologically experienced as ugly, undesirable and dangerous, even though the older person may look as good as ever, or better.

The Negative Body Image

Most people do not succumb to complete breakdowns because of this. Rather, they suffer silently and secretly through the many mini-crises which cause disturbance of their body image, such as dentures, hearing aid, bifocals, or arthritic interference with tennis. Unconsciously, the older person will incorporate each change into the body image as a "hallmark" of old age, and respond accordingly. Many of the personality changes we attribute to aging—withdrawal, irascibility, resentment—are really a person's defenses against anticipated rejection by others, and eventually become self-rejection. This, plus a body that cannot be trusted is hardly conducive to "swinging."

The negative body image is so subtle that even healthy, happy, normally functioning older people may have it and not know it. It strikes only when a person's defenses are down. If you are over sixty, there's an easy test to prove it to yourself.

Just take a pencil and a piece of paper and draw a picture of a person. Do this before reading further.

You may be astonished at what comes out, if anything at all does. Many older people are so blocked about their body image that they cannot produce more than a stick drawing.

For those who can draw, the results may be startling, even shocking. Some of the most distinguished senior citizens, who are still functioning in high gear and who still look superb, produce drawings indistinguishable from those of mental patients who have been institutionalized for years. The people they draw may be tiny and distorted or vague and formless, oozing all over or off the page. Parts may be exaggerated or left out entirely, or so bizarre the person who drew the picture can hardly believe it.

One man in his seventies drew a large outline figure whose torso was an empty square with a glaring interruption of line in the genital area and an enormous phallic necktie on the otherwise unadorned body. Another in his seventies drew a meticulous picture of an idealized male, in sartorial splendor, but gave the arms neat circular endings as if the hands had been hacked off at the wrists.

Even accomplished artists over sixty show little telltale signs of an unconscious, negative body image in their drawings: a suspiciously darkened line here, a quirk of expression there, a significant omission. A picture drawn in profile, facing outward in the left hand corner of a page, tells you something about a person, does it not?

What about you?

Your picture came out pretty good, did it? No distortions, no omissions, no suspicious lines or details? No signs of self-rejection, no body-image disturbances? Well, keep it that way! Remember, body-image problems come up when our defenses are down. So when the dentist tells you that crown will have to be replaced with a bridge or, more seriously, when there is illness or loss, make sure you face the real issues instead of displacing your feelings on your body image.

The Body Is Willing But the Mind Isn't

This is an unexpected and unwelcome switch now that society has finally begun to recognize the sexual needs of older people. One suggestion made quite seriously in contemporary medical literature is to promote polygamy among the smaller number of males over sixty so that the longer-lived women can be assured of sexual partners.

But the sad fact remains that even with sexual partners available, older people may find themselves unloved sexually because they think of themselves as unlovable. A negative body image can obliterate the sex drive, and even the drive for human contact.

Even if a person swallows shame and shyness and bravely makes a try, chances are he or she will succumb to anger and withdrawal at the very first rebuff, sometimes with disastrous results. One swinging bachelor had his first heart attack and a major depression after he was given his first brush-off at age seventy. At least he claimed it was his first. No doubt he survived through more than a few rejections during his long, active sexual career, but the crucial seventieth birthday, and a negative body image forming within him rendered his ego so fragile that this one untimely rebuff sent him over the edge.

For those lucky few who are blissfully unmindful of their vein-laced thighs and stomach bulges—and what is even luckier, of the derisive remarks of resentful peers—there are the many who wear long sleeves to hide flab, or turtlenecks on the hottest days, and who shrink with embarrassment when approached for just a friendly kiss.

Who says we become tougher as we mature? Past sixty, we are as psychologically vunerable as we were in adolescence. We again have creaking joints, sudden reflexes, recalcitrant muscles. We panic at the thought of rejection, we hide in a world of fantasy.

It takes more than sex to make a person over sixty sexy. It takes self-acceptance and acceptance of the others over sixty. Too often we accept ourselves after sixty by disassociating from the others—*they* are old. Which still leaves us out in left field, without partners!

Fortunately, the longer we live, the more libido we accrue in the good old Freudian sense. Even without direct sexual outlets, the sex drive is a healthy, energizing life force that can infiltrate all kinds of activities and involvements with joy and zest. We are capable of "libidinizing" anything from shuffleboard to mathematics. But by focusing obsessively on the sex act alone, we can cut off other good possibilities and the sex act as well.

Sex and Senility

It is possible that if older people were encouraged to find sexual release in fantasy or otherwise, and taught how to if necessary, most senility might be eradicated. As it is, the *functioning* lifetime is increasing dramatically in this age of sexual permissiveness. Twenty-five years ago, the average age in the old folks home was in the mid-fifties; today it is in the mid-eighties.

People no longer go to the nursing home to wait for death. They end up there shortly before death, although we tend to focus on the painful details of that sad end and overlook the fact that more and more older people are capable of really living until the end. After all, only about five percent of us end up in the nursing home; the rest of us die in bed, at the office, or on the golf course.

But "senior liberation" is just beginning. Seldom is sex therapy offered to the disoriented, confused senile person, even though the topic of sex comes up explicitly and regularly in whatever psychotherapy is offered to older persons—and even though, when sex is finally discussed, it is usually the turning point toward recovery.

Mrs. S., age eighty, came complete with the diagnosis of chronic brain syndrome to a mental health clinic for older people. The fact that such a "hopeless" case was even accepted for treatment represents a big advance in our thinking. As Mrs. S. groped her way back from disorientation and confusion to depression and panic, and finally to stability, it turned out that she had been carrying a torch for a certain gentleman all of her adult life. They had been engaged many years before, when he jilted her to marry someone else.

Her own marriage did not work out, but she nevertheless led a contented life after her divorce, working at interesting jobs, traveling, enjoying friendships, and surviving until eighty without any major mishaps. This probably would have continued had she not received a letter from her first love, out of the blue, telling her he was now widowed, would be visiting in her town, and wanted to have dinner.

They met, had dinner, and that was it: he went his way. Shortly, Mrs. S. became depressed and fearful. She lost her appetite and finally her mind, as she put it. The woman later insisted that she had a nervous breakdown because her eightieth birthday made her feel old and "finished." This was probably true. But her cure came about only after she had worked through her feelings of sexual frustration and rejection.

Mr. B., age sixty four, an occasionally employed typographer, blacked out one day and was rushed to the hospital, where it was discovered he had dangerously high blood pressure. While there, he was confused and disoriented and had some difficulty speaking, but he recovered fairly quickly. Psychological testing showed there had been no impairment of mental faculties; in fact, Mr. B. had a surprisingly high I.Q.

His wife, however, insisted that her husband remain in the hospital, because according to her, he had memory loss and other sign of "senility." Mr. B. did not seem in any hurry to leave either. They were referred to marital counseling, where it was revealed that their marriage had been in name only since their last child was born some twenty-five years earlier. Mrs. B. claimed not to be interested in sex, staying in the marriage "for the sake of the children." She supported the family as well as running the home.

Mr. B. always did what he was told and stayed out of her way. But now his possible "little stroke" scared his wife. The last thing she wanted was to take care of a senile spouse after she was finally freed from her duties as a mother.

Actually, Mr. B. did oblige by showing some signs of "senility," and might have ended up in a nursing home had the marital counselor not suggested another solution: divorce. The couple readily agreed. His blood pressure subsided, and according to her own statement, she began to "live for the first time in my life."

Is it possible that older people opt for "senility" rather than face their suppressed sexual conflicts, their rage, and other overwhelming emotions? In many cases, it certainly seems so. A change in the sexual balance between husband and wife may cause one or the other to retreat into memory loss or confusion or other symptoms of deterioration.

One vigorous man in his early seventies developed "memory loss" as an excuse to give up his lucrative contracting business, which bored him, and his mistress, who also did. When this did not work with her, he became impotent and ended the affair that way. His recovery from both came about when he persuaded his wife, a successful, practicing physician and lifelong ego-threat to him, to retire with him to Arizona. There he is enjoying golf, bridge, and saunas—though one wonders what is happening to his wife.

The Late-Blooming Homosexual

Homosexual fantasies occur in older heterosexuals just as they do in younger ones. These fantasies are not abnormal but are part of the "universal unconscious." They add spice to sexual fantasies and can alleviate the stale marriage syndrome.

Sudden, overwhelming homosexual impulses, however, are quite a different story, especially if acted upon. There can be devastating effects on family, friends, and above all on the older person himself or herself. This type of alien, compulsive homosexual drive usually indicates panic related to an entirely different life-crisis, such as illness, death or financial loss. It arises from guilt and fear and is used to punish and degrade the self, which has been rejected because of the person's inability to accept his natural aging.

However, there are also instances of homosexuality in older age which represent a voluntary "coming out of the closet" because the individual now feels safe and secure enough to do so. Homosexuality may reflect a conscious choice of a new sexual lifestyle among women so inclined, as the ranks of men thin out. It may evolve quite naturally out of the friendship, trust, and affection which develop among surviving women in older age groups.

Is homosexuality recommended as a solution to loneliness in older age? If one is consciously consenting, homosexuality as a free choice certainly cannot hurt. But if there is panic, denial of reality, and guilt, homosexuality is a sickness rather than a sexual release. It may even cause suicide.

One distinguished gentleman made repeated suicide attempts for no apparent reason, denying he was depressed or even discontent. The suicidal impulse, he said, simply came upon him.

Psychological testing revealed his unconscious was crowded with severely repressed homosexual fantasies. Apparently, whenever there was an overload of these fantasies, he experienced a breakthrough of homosexual impulse—against which he had no defense but suicide.

A man who has been a lifelong homosexual, on the other hand, may find his homosexuality an advantage in dealing with the old-age crisis, at least according to an intensive study of the homosexual community in New York City. Investigators, found that male homosexuals experience a major age crisis much earlier in life, and therefore have more time to build up compensations for loneliness and rejection. Further, having never assumed the traditional male role in American society, they do not have to face the loss of masculinity and usefulness which affects so many men after retirement.

Swinging after Sixty? Suit Yourself

This seems to be an era where anything goes, and the present generation over age sixty wrote the book on it. In a way, it is almost as if the times are catching up with them instead of the other way around. And their behavior proves it: there are very few "old" people today.

Many who are old are not so because of their age, but because of hang-ups which make old age an easier "out." Sex can be a casualty of unresolved conflict at any age. Resolve the conflict, and to swing or not to swing becomes a personal affair—and nobody else's business.

Chapter Nine

What Kind of Old Person Will You Be?

"We must always change, renew, rejuvenate ourselves ... otherwise we harden."

Goethe

Learn Your AQ (Aging Quotient)

You are invited to take a "test" to learn about your attitudes towards aging: it is the Oberleder Attitude Scale. Just follow the instructions, read each statement carefully, and answer each one. If you are not absolutely sure how you want to answer, answer anyway in the direction you feel. You probably will not have any difficulty making up your mind.

Scoring instructions follow the test. The test contains twenty five statements. After each statement circle:

(A) If you agree with it completely.
(a) If you agree with it, but with some reservations.
(D) If you disagree with it, but only slightly.
(d) If you disagree with the statement strongly.

1. The older you get, the more set in your ways you become . . . . A a d D
2. Old age can be said to begin around 60 or 65 . . . . A a d D
3. Old people too often like to meddle in other people's business . . . . A a d D
4. Older people become grouchy and stubborn with the years . . . . A a d D
5. Old people can, and are, learning new things all the time . . . . A a d D
6. Older people cannot be expected to lead a completely full or satisfying life . . . . A a d D
7. As you grow older, you become less and less useful . . . . A a d D
8. People get shorter as they grow older . . . . A a d D
9. You can't teach an old dog new tricks . . . . A a d D
10. Old people would prefer to have some kind of work to do . . . . A a d D
11. Special housing projects for just old people is not a good idea, but the city should reserve apartments in the regular housing projects for old people. That way, people of all ages are together . . . . A a d D
12. It is usually a mistake for people over 65 to marry . . . . A a d D
13. A person is really glad to retire from work at 65 or 70 . . . . A a d D
14. Old people usually don't talk very much . . . . A a d D
15. Old people are adjusting to new conditions all the time, and are doing it easily . . . . A a d D
16. There should be special radio and TV programs for older folks . . . . A a d D
17. Older people should enroll in classes which train them for a new kind of work . . A a d D
18. Old people like to boss everybody . . A a d D

19. Older people should let the others do the work and get the credit .... A a d D
20. As you grow older you must expect to depend on others .... A a d D
21. People should always try for something better, no matter how old they are .... A a d D
22. Old people prefer to be with people their own age .... A a d D
23. Old people need special foods ...... A a d D
24. Physical exercise of some kind is good for you as you grow older .... A a d D
25. Trying to learn a new job in older age strikes me as a little silly .... A a d D

Scoring Key

(Your score is the total number of points circled.)

Score one (1) point if you have circled

Item		Item	
1.	A or a	14.	D or d
2.	A or a	15.	D or d
3.	A or a	16.	A or a
4.	A or a	17.	D or d
5.	D or d	18.	A or a
6.	A or a	19.	A or a
7.	A or a	20.	A or a
8.	A or a	21.	A or a
9.	A or a	22.	A or a
10.	D or d	23.	A or a
11.	D or d	24.	D or d
12.	A or a	25.	A or a
13.	A or a		_____ Total score

What Does Your Score Mean?

As you have guessed, this test measures the degree to which you accept or reject some of the stereotypes connected with aging. It also determines whether your attitudes are positive or negative in respect to aging.

For instance, if you agreed with item 9 ("You can't teach an old dog new tricks"), it would indicate that you accept this stereotype as true. If you accept enough stereotypes (this would be reflected in the *higher scores*), it would also indicate that you have somewhat negative attitudes toward aging and old people.

If, on the other hand, you refuse to accept the stereotype and disagree with item 9, along with others that represent sterotypes, and if you agree with the more positive statements, such as item 5 ("Old people can, and are, learning new things all the time"), this will be reflected in the *lower scores*. It means your attitudes toward aging and old people are generally positive, accepting, and optimistic.

Who will adjust better to aging, low scorers or high scorers? Generally, scores between 4 and 13 indicate a good adjustment to aging if by adjustment we mean: a person who is cheerful, realistic, cooperative, able to get along with others, socially active, and yet able to enjoy and pursue individual interests. Such people do not lose their tempers easily, they accept the negative aspects of aging "philosophically," and avoid disruptive situations skillfully without being evasive or submissive.

People with scores upwards of 15 tend to report more problems in adjustment to aging, and are often problems to their friends and relatives as well. They may be critical of others, complaining and demanding; or they may be self-centered and insensitive to others. People who are depressed and withdrawn also tend to have higher scores.

Attitudes and Adjustment

Your attitudes determine how you will respond to a given situation. More than that, they determine how you will perceive a situation, even before you do anything about it. Reality itself may have very little to do with your attitudes—and consequently with your reactions.

There's a story about a man who was having one of those days when everything goes wrong and finally climaxed with a flat tire on his car. Fuming, he went next door to borrow a jack from his neighbor. On the way, he remembered some arguments he had had with the neighbor, and also that he had forgotten to return his lawn mower. When the neighbor opened his door, our man yelled, "You can keep your damn jack!" and turned and left.

Your attitudes toward aging are the most crucial factor in your adjustment to aging, as well as the most difficult to change. If you had a high score on the test, you should consider seriously changing your attitudes—no matter how difficult it may be to do so.

Which attitudes are the worst? Those that are both critical and defeatist. On the questionnaire they are represented by statements like, "Old people too often like to meddle in other people's business" and "Old people like to boss everybody." They not only put the old person down, they don't leave any hope for improvement.

The best attitudes are those that represent a vigorous, positive stand: "Old people are adjusting to new conditions all the time and are doing it easily"; "Physical exercise of some kind is good for you as you grow older."

The questionnaire has been used in many different settings, for many different purposes, and has proven reliable in predicting adjustment both to aging and to older people. In institutions for the elderly, low-scorers manage to adjust well while high-scorers often become "management problems." In hospital training programs, student nurses and other personnel who are low-scorers do well with the elderly patients, while the high-scorers have to be assigned elsewhere.

High-scorers on the questionnaire also turn out to be "authoritarian," "rigid," "prejudiced," and "opinionated" on other tests of personality.

And when people are ill they will score higher on this questionnaire than when well, regardless of age. Illness makes everybody feel "old" in the stereotyped sense of the word, and that shows up on the high score. Later on, when there is recovery from illness, scores will go down as spirits rise and the patient takes a more positive, optimistic point of view.

This questionnaire is one test where it pays to have a low score.

Scores at the Extreme Ends

There are people who score 0 and 1 or 2 and others who score as high as 25 on the questionnaire. They are people who either see nothing bad about aging, or nothing good about it. They are not as different from each other as you might think—in fact they are very much alike.

The only difference between them is that the low-scorers use "denial" while the high scorers use "dissociation." Both distort the truth about their own aging, and both adjust well to being old.

Low-scorers or "deniers" take a positive stand on everything, which is all to the good in older age. Sometimes there is concern that deniers may overlook some conditions that require treatment because they are so positive about everything and refuse to recognize illness or other problems.

However, you don't really have to worry about them. They are so determined to be in tip-top shape that they take very good care of themselves. They live right, eat right, and enjoy life. They are not likely to let a problem get the better of them.

High-scorers who see nothing good about aging and who see old people as all bad manage to survive to very old age by dissociating themselves from aging altogether. That is, psychologically. Very often they are the ones who do good works for other older people and make up the bulk of the various volunteer services. Bless them for it!

One woman resident of a retirement home who scored 24 on the questionnaire by agreeing with all the negative stereotypes and disagreeing with the positive statements, wrote in the margin, "These are not necessarily my sentiments, but merely my observations."

This particular woman, by the way, won $64,000 on a TV quiz program at the age of seventy-eight and lived out her final years caring for the others—taking them for walks, reading to them, writing letters for them, and the like. She was a delightful, enchanting woman, and it is a fact that you never thought of her age when you were with her.

Nor did one mind that she was opinionated and more than a bit authoritarian.

It is a form of adjustment to refuse to accept old age for yourself, or to deny that it exists. What you are doing is *reversing the negative expectancy*. But in order to get away with it you must be conflict-free—and very few of us are.

It is better for most of us to maintain a positive stance while facing our issues squarely. Of course, a little denial is good for the soul occasionally, and so long as we don't lose sight of reality. Most important is that we remain *flexible*—ready to change. There is evidence that people who cling to "tradition" have more problems with aging than their more daring brothers and sisters.

Is it true that, "the older you get, the more set in your ways you become?" That's the biggest myth of all. If you're set in your ways, you were that way to begin with. And it's about time you changed!

Who Wants to Be Old?

Most people want to live a long time but few people want to be "old." So how do they handle it? They think of themselves as "middle-aged." In one study, large numbers of people *over age eighty five* who were asked to identify themselves in terms of age checked off "middle-aged."

People who were willing to label themselves "old" or "elderly" actually had a higher mortality rate, and many did not live until the restudy which took place ten years later.

So denial of aging is not only good for the soul, it helps you live longer.

But were these people really denying their *age?* No, they admitted their age. They merely rejected the age-designation of "old," and the negative stereotypes associated with being old. They wished to be identified by how they felt about themselves, and not by society's label.

When do people think they are "old"? Only when something happens to alter their lifestyle downward. Sickness, widowhood, loss of independence, reduced income—*entrapment*: it is only when people feel trapped, without hope of escape, that they feel "old."

Most of us weather the downward changes that inevitably occur with aging unless they hit us all at once. In recent times, more opportunities have developed for older people to fight entrapment. We are entering older age with more going for us and more ways of compensating and substituting for losses as they occur.

Of course, the negative, dreary social myths about aging persist, but there is evidence that even this may have an advantage. When older people today compare themselves with the myths, they are delighted to see how much better off they are.

And the last thing they want to do is identify with being "Old." So "middle-aged" we are, until the end—or shortly before. That's what the studies show and that's the way it will probably be until society makes some changes in its concept of being old.

"Old Is Beautiful"

As older people begin to accept themselves, a new sense of power is developing. They remain masters of their own lives, especially in communities that permit independent living and positive communication and interaction among older people. They no longer think of themselves as "second-class" citizens in comparison with young people. According to sociologists, a "subculture of age" is forming.

From such a subculture we can hope for an "aging group consciousness" and an "aging group pride." As older people think of themselves as a "group," as a "subculture," they can build a new and more positive social world for themselves.

This is already happening in many retirement communities where the studies show much higher morale, much more positive interaction and much more willingness to identify with an older age group than in the general community.

The problem is, however, that even though people feel better about themselves, are rarely lonely, and feel needed and useful in these age-segregated communities, they are nevertheless *retreatist* communities. People chose to be there to avoid the negative aspects of the broader community.

The sociologists had hoped that as the older person's self-image became more positive and as group identity developed, the aging would become more activist using *group power* in a way that would change society's outmoded and defeatist ideas about aging.

This has not yet happened, at least in retirement communities, which still serve as "havens" where the older person can retreat and heal wounds gotten in the course of social aging. But still, the age-segregated community offers the best possibility for the restoration of power to the older person. Each five-year interval brings another kind of "retiree" to the age-segregated community; and as the aging picture continues to change, the chances are that the sociologists' prediction of "More Power for the (Aging) People!" in general will come about.

Not All Change Is Good

An eye doctor I know said he could always tell when his patients turn forty. That is when they get presbyopia—farsightedness.

Naturally, there'll be some changes as you grow older, and it would take some doing to convince you that they are for the best. But many probably have some place in the natural course of human development and for all we know these natural changes may be better than the alternative.

As we have seen, many of the changes associated with aging are gross exaggerations of what nature intended, and many are not due to aging at all. Generally speaking, our adjustment to aging will depend on how we can match each new change to our already established expectations; is it as bad or worse than we expected, and how we can fit it into our lifestyle? Arthritis interferes with hiking—but not with bicycling and swimming.

The kind of old person you will be depends on how well you compensate for changes to maintain the pleasure-balance of your life. Low-scorers on the questionnaire have the advantage over high-scorers by far.

So, what kinds of changes can you expect? Visual changes for sure. But after the first impact, farsightedness usually levels off for about twenty years, changing again at about age sixty. After sixty there may be more difficulty in discriminating details and "dark adaptation" may decrease somewhat. Almost all the changes that take place naturally and are not exaggerated by environmental insults can be compensated for naturally, or with the aid of eyeglasses, eye exercises, and the like. Even cataracts are a curable disease for the vast majority who get them.

Psychological factors are crucial elements in how we adapt to these natural changes. If we are obsessed with them, if we are infuriated, if they affect our personality and behavior, then of course they will destroy us. Highscorers beware!

And yes, there may be some hearing loss, particularly after age sixty-five and particularly for high-pitched sounds. Because of it, older people may have more trouble identifying what they hear. They will be especially penalized when speech is too rapid, or garbled, or mechanically distorted as on the TV and the radio. If you have an answering machine on your telephone, be sure your announcement is clear and slow so that it can be easily comprehended by your elderly callers. It doesn't hurt to repeat the key words, either.

Psychological factors, especially tension and anxiety, will exaggerate deafness. And there is another problem. Deafness is an isolating handicap, even more so than poor vision. The hard-of-hearing sometimes get out of the habit of paying attention. The old observation, "They hear what they want to hear" has a good deal of truth in it. But it does not make for good adjustment in older age.

We've included hearing loss as a natural change with age because over 50 percent of people over sixty-five have it to some degree. But environmental factors exercise a profound influence on hearing, especially in respect to noise and other forms of hearing shock. The fact stands that hearing loss occurs more in the Western world. So perhaps we should think in terms of preventing hearing loss, as well as compensating for it.

What are some of the other changes? Wrinkles, thinning hair, thinning bones, muscle weakness, sickness? No, these are not changes that are necessarily due to aging. Even sickness. According to a medical saying, "There are no illnesses peculiar to old age, and none from which it is free."

True, older age may increase your chances of getting all these things but it does not guarantee that you will. Your attitudes toward aging will be the determining factor. Recent studies are beginning to show that even declining health does not affect the life-satisfaction of the modern older person, who is flexible and positive in his outlook. High-scorers, you have a lot to learn from the low-scorers!

Your Unconscious Attitudes

The attitude questionnaire revealed your conscious attitudes. But what about your unconscious attitudes? Well, you should obtain quite a bit of information about those from the other "tests" included in this book. What about the picture of a person you drew? Was it large, clear, facing front, drawn with firm lines?

Never mind that it was not a work of art. The larger drawings have been associated with higher intelligence, unless of course they are just big, vague, formless shapes. But if it is well-detailed and the lines are strong, you've got a good mind working for you. And a front-face position reflects how you yourself face the world—ready to meet it, with nothing to hide. You should have scored low on the questionnaire. If you didn't, then there still may be a few wrinkles in your attitudes towards aging. Nothing to worry about, you'll be able to handle it.

But wait, do you have some extra dark lines here and there that seem to stand out from the rest? Extra shading in spots? These will have to be analyzed. They represent repressed feelings—usually aggressive or sexual, depending on where they are. Too much repression, as we already know, is not good for adjustment, especially to aging. You might want to do something about identifying those repressed feelings. Remember you don't have to act on them, just learn what they are and how they affect your conscious attitudes. People who cling to the stereotypes and have generally negative attitudes towards old people are probably displacing their negative feelings about themselves on others.

Or was your drawing very small and off to one side? No need to be so shy and resentful. Come and join the rest of us, we're all in the same boat, and as we've been saying all along, there's strength in numbers.

What? You couldn't even draw a whole person, only a head? That means your mind won't have anything to do with the rest of you; your mind and body each go their separate ways. It's sort of a combination of impulsivity and inhibition, and many old people are just like that: they do the most outrageous things, and yet they're bland and innocent when confronted with their acts. Don't fall into that trap: get to know your *whole* self.

Is your drawing a mess, really terrible? Well, you may be embracing old age too soon, or you may be depressed. Anyway, even though you're willing to accept old age (maybe too willingly), you don't really like it. You're one of the high-scorers who should do something about changing your attitudes towards aging —pronto.

But wait! Don't throw that picture away. First make up a little story about it by answering the following questions.

1. What's the person you drew doing?
2. How old is he or she?
3. Is the person married?
4. Does he or she have children? What ages? Girls? Boys?
5. With whom does the person live?
6. To whom is he or she most attached?
7. Does he or she have brothers or sisters?
8. What sort of work does the person do?
9. How much schooling has the person had?
10. What are her or his ambitions?
11. Is the person smart?
12. Strong?
13. Healthy?
14. Good-looking?
15. What is the best part of the person?
16. The worst part?
17. What's on his or her mind?
18. What are this person's fears?
19. What gets her or him angry?
20. What does he or she wish for the most?
21. Is the person sad or happy?
22. Happier alone or with other people?
23. What do people say about this person?
24. Does the person trust people?
25. Is he or she afraid of people?

Give the story an ending. Now read it over, with an open mind.

No Scores—Just Insights

There are no scores on that Tell-a-Story Test, just information about yourself, your frustrations and satisfactions. You may discover how you really feel about someone close to you, or you may have answered the questions facetiously to avoid finding out about yourself. Okay, it's good to know that too, isn't it?

There were no scores on the Hidden Word Test either. But if you missed out on words like "mother," "will," "spouse," and "death," that tells you something, and not necessarily that you have serious problems in those four cases. Rather, you tend to put things out of your mind when they are bothersome. And when you do, it interferes with your functioning, in this case memory.

This tendency to put disturbing thoughts out of mind may affect your conscious attitudes toward aging. Both high-scorers and low-scorers do it. Just don't let it interfere with your functioning too much. Thought-blocking can be dangerous to your mental health.

Chapter Ten

Meet the New Elderly

"You have to be old before you can enjoy being young in spirit."

Malcolm S. Forbes

"I'm Too Young to Sit Around"

So says an eighty-six-year-old man interviewed in a recent Harris Poll study of Americans over sixty-five, called "The Myth and Reality of Aging in America."

This survey once again proves that the myth and reality of aging are very different from each other—and that younger people's ideas about aging are very different from the reality of aging as experienced by the elderly themselves.

In reality, older people claim that they are very much better off than they ever expected to be. It seems, according to the study, that "the picture drawn in the public's mind of old age and its problems is a gross distortion of what older people say they experience personally."

What is the reality according to older people themselves? They are healthier, better off financially, and live longer than ever before. They are also better educated and more independent, both in spirit and lifestyle. If the young could be made to fully realize this it would no doubt ease their consciences and sense of "burden" about older people, especially their parents, and relieve fears about their own aging. It would also ease older people's guilt about their own high spirits.

Only one person in 10, the survey showed, felt that older age turned out worse than expected. And the problems were due to race, poverty or lack of education rather than age itself. This study and others prove that to cure the problems of aging, one must focus on problems that are entirely separate from aging.

The Problems of Today's Elderly

They are the same as everybody else's. Given a list of problems to evaluate, the elderly placed them in this order of importance:

- Not enough money
- Loneliness
- Not feeling needed
- Fear of crime
- Poor health
- Not enough job opportunities
- Not enough medical care
- Not enough to do to keep busy
- Not enough friends
- Not enough education
- Not enough clothing

People under and over sixty-five ranked these problems similarly, except that older people were more worried about poor health, crime, and a lack of job opportunities. But none of the problems were exclusive to aging—all are problems of our society as a whole.

The investigators warned that the persisting myth of the elderly being an economically and socially deprived group not only generates guilt and pity among the young, but actually prevents young people from appreciating the talents and energies of older people. In addition, it makes them fear their own aging as well.

An example of this appears in an article written by a worried daughter who was so fearful that her parent would have an emergency in the middle of the night that she frequently checked the airlines to be sure she could get there on time. The writer saw her parents not only as a "problem" but as her problem exclusively. She worried about the "call," should it come on a holiday, or during a blizzard when no flights would be available. For her the problem of aging parents outstripped childrearing, marital and personal problems.

Some young people may need the aging myths as some older people do: to avoid facing their real day-to-day problems. And there might be something else, too: as this writer said, "Facing their death means facing our own. Once our parents go, we're next in line."

Another article entitled "The Elderly Beached by Life's Ebbing Tide," pitied the older population who live in Miami Beach. The writer was apparently unaware of the fact that three out of four people over sixty-five said that life was as interesting as ever and over half expected it to be even better in the future. What stayed with him were "those awful words from the hit record, 'Hope I Die Before I Get Old!'"

Whom Are We Worried About?

Most Americans sixty-five and older are healthy, self-supporting, own their homes and have paid off the mortgage.

They're not complaining, except about crime. But here their fears may be exaggerated, for as recent studies show, the elderly are *less* victimized by crime than other age groups.

They are the second-fastest-growing age group, having reached almost 25 million in 1979 and are projected to reach well over 30 million by the year 2000. They are surpassed by the 18-to-44-year group only by a fraction of a percent.

Those over sixty-five are more educated and less foreign-born than ever before; they are more like everyone else, which means no great social adjustments are required of them.

They are in familiar territory. Why shouldn't they be happy? Usually, the ones who are not are in poor health or have a spouse who is. Most have a strong image of self-reliance, and despite retirement laws, at least a fourth of them are still working.

Generally, the "New Elderly" see themselves in a favorable light. They don't accept the stereotypes, at least not for themselves: they don't feel they have to apologize for their age; they describe themselves as open-minded, adaptable, warm, and alert; they think they are as intelligent as they ever were and probably wiser. They take steps to preserve their memory and don't panic when it sometimes fails them. They know how to pace themselves.

Here's what some of them say:

"I still don't feel old, even at seventy-seven. I realize that I look old and I have occasional pain, but since anyone can have pain that doesn't mean that I am old. I must have passed middle age a long time ago without noticing it."

"I really don't give much thought to growing old and certainly am not intimidated by it."

"Age doesn't matter; maybe some day I'll feel old, but it hasn't happened yet."

"So here we are (at eighty) and feeling much the same."

"At sixty-five, I felt old, anticipating possible physical incapacity. Now, five years later ... I feel younger than I did at sixty."

"It was the concern of my children about my being alone that caused me ... to move to the (retirement) village. After refusing to live with them or take an apartment near them. . . I felt I owed it to them to relieve their worries about me."

"I resent and always have, the implication that the elderly are a disagreeable burden, foisted on the rest of the population ... when older people are treated as people, they contribute a full share and carry their own weight."

"I am going to consciously plan to get the most out of every day ... acquire more knowledge ... find ways to contribute to society ... laugh more ... successfully adapt to changes ... without fear or worry about the future..."

"Now I come to the most important suggestion ... suicide kits for the intellectually competent elderly to be available for terminal cancer or other terminal illness... To me it would be a tremendous comfort to have a pill stored safely in the drawer ... I'd take it as casually as I'd brush my teeth..."

"Old age has removed any fear of death. Relatives and close friends have died. If they could encompass it, so can we."

Most of these statements were made by people upwards of seventy five. They were of the higher socioeconomic bracket, and many were professionals. As the Harris Poll investigators said, "The negative stereotype of the aged vanishes when the old are educated, affluent, and 'healthy.'"

It is also important to remember the converse of that statement. When people are uneducated, poor, and ill, they become old before their time. They not only fit the negative view of aging, they probably cause it.

Fortunately, the number of older people who are under the poverty line has decreased considerably —from 30 percent in 1965 to 14 percent in 1980. Even that is too high a number of course, but it is expected to continue to drop as the young and middle-aged of today grow older and reap benefits from longer term Social Security and pensions which the elderly now do not have.

The "Age-Irrelevant Society"

That's what gerontologist Bernice Neugarten calls it. Indeed, what else can one call a society which, as she points out, is not surprised by a twenty-two-year-old mayor, a twenty-nine-year-old university president, and a seventy-year-old college freshman!

Some time ago, when it was suggested that women marry men eight to ten years younger than themselves in order to avoid being widows, they merely laughed.

Today they *do* it. And often the men are fifteen and twenty years younger! Of course, this is still not as acceptable as men marrying women twenty and thirty years younger, but it's happening more and more. Society's age attitudes are shifting.

Neugarten believes the cult of youth is fading fast in this country and that in another decade or two it will be gone altogether. One reason for it, she believes, is sheer numbers. One out of every ten persons is over sixty-five, and people upwards of eighty are doing things that would not have been dreamed of thirty years ago.

Nobody says, "act your age" anymore. Older people switch careers, go back to school, marry, divorce, and remarry. A man can become a father at the same time he becomes a grandfather.

Neugarten isn't necessarily recommending all this, but she is pointing out that "older people feel younger today." They marvel at how much different they are from their parents who were considered "old" at their age.

Even grandparents have moved down a generation, and great-grandparents have come to take their place. Today, many grandparents are working. On their days off, they are more likely to be playmates rather than authority figures to their grandchildren. (A TV commercial shows grandma taking little Billy horseback riding as the two giggle and tease each other at a pretty fast trot.) It's now up to great-grandparents to provide the wise, authoritarian figure of former days.

Of course, not all grandparents can get away with being playmates. An article entitled, "Recycling Grandparents as Parents" in the *Los Angeles Times* describes how some must pitch in as parents to take care of orphaned grandchildren, or offspring of divorced sons and daughters, or they fill in for working parents.

Regardless of the reason, it is an arrangement more of necessity than choice, and it is a very fast-developing trend. Do grandparents like it? Some are delighted, to be sure, but large numbers are dismayed. Although the grandchildren, even those of college age, are more comfortable confiding in their grandparents than they are in their parents.

"You're not old," said one. "You have wrinkles on your skin, but you are not wrinkled inside."

Another explained, "When you live with your mother and your grandparents, your mom becomes a child. She's like an older sister more than a mother."

Now, with the increase of divorce, a new type of grandparent has entered the picture, the step-grandparents. Older people may find themselves faced with several sets of grandchildren to whom they are not related at all, and social workers fear this may create problems. But the likelihood is that step-grandparents will solve more problems than they will create, motivated as they will be to maintain relationships with their own grandchildren.

Exit the "Nuclear" Family

Enter the extended family—or to be more precise, reenter the extended family. The days of mother, father, and 2.6 children are over, at least for the time being. The days of the four-generation family are here. Finding it too expensive to live alone, a young couple with children is often forced to return to the parental home. And a divorced parent with children to raise may have no choice in the matter: he or she must go to work. Grandma and grandpa to the rescue!

Today's elderly may be a vital factor in the lives of the young people around them—providing money, emotional support, advice, housekeeping, childrearing, chauffering, everything a parent does.

Although problems can result from this kind of rescue work, most grandparents seem to take it in stride. The traditional "differences" between the generations does not seem to interfere so much anymore, if they exist at all. Young and old share many of the same ideas and experiences, making both more sympathetic and cooperative. The sharing of childrearing chores for example, has an equalizing effect in that it keeps grandparents young in outlook. They have to be—if they aren't, a grandchild lets them know it soon enough.

Do the grandchildren benefit from an "extended" family? Immeasurably. Not only are they exposed to more experiences, more intimacies, more supportive relationships (bound to create inner security and self-confidence), but they develop awareness and appreciation of the older person. They are not likely to fear their own aging under such circumstances. Thus, a major source of psychological "hang-ups" is automatically removed.

Do grandparents benefit from the extended family? Not necessarily. It is not like the old days when the family hearth was the old person's final resting place. The New Elderly do not suffer from the empty nest syndrome. When the children grow up and get out, they are quick to follow. Called back from the golf course or camping trip, grandparents may not be all that tickled about it. "Recycled parenthood isn't what it's cracked up to be," states one.

But of course, they'll do it.

To Work or Not to Work

The idea of retirement is a modern-day, machine-age concept. It was born suddenly in the 20th century, when it was thought that assembly lines would render the worker obsolete.

But what wasn't counted on was the "graying of America": the modern worker is an older worker. And since the labor pool needs labor, the concept of retirement may disappear as suddenly as it was born.

Those who really want to retire, the blue-collar and clerical workers whose jobs are dull, leave a big vacuum which has to be filled. Professionals are reluctant to retire as a rule, and increasing numbers of them do not have to do so. Those who are caught by mandatory retirement laws are often retired and rehired elsewhere immediately afterward. In any case, they do not leave a vacuum, because their jobs are desirable and people compete for them.

Thus, the New Elderly facing a *need* to work rather than a choice, due to inflation, boredom, and personal energy build-up, are taking the jobs others do not want: selling, cashier work, stenography, housekeeping, nursing, repair work, bookkeeping, and clerical work.

Are they bored? Usually not, because this is the sort of thing they were used to earlier in their lives in the pre-electric typewriter days. Older workers value and appreciate work, and except in jobs requiring very fast reaction times, they do as well, and often better than younger workers. Accuracy and consistency of output *increase* with age. Older workers have lower job turnover rates because they are more stable individuals. They have less accidents because they are more careful. They have less absenteeism because they are more dedicated. And they are more experienced than younger workers.

Most of them really want to work, too—as long as they are able. Many have retired against their will, and those who wanted to retire may find they need money. Increasingly, they are going into "second careers," and doing an entirely different kind of work than before. A physician became a travel agent; a former dress manufacturer became a bank teller in his retirement community. Countless women, married and widowed, have gone to work after age seventy-two when their Social Security payments are no longer jeopardized. This includes women who have never worked before.

More and more older people are entering the work force in both full-time and part-time employment. All the surveys indicate that it is really what they want to do. It makes them a part of the times.

Getting the Most from the Older Worker

In a most important study, researchers James L. Fozard and Samuel J. Popkin show that environments should be designed to accommodate the changing needs of adults as they grow older—to keep them functioning at optimal levels.

We know that the working population, like the general population, will become increasingly older. We know what changes can be expected to occur in the course of normal aging. We have the information, and the technology. Now, it is simply a matter of studying workers of all ages and designing environments responsive to their needs.

Besides workplace decorating, coffee breaks, background music, and incentives are all examples of environmental planning for the increased efficiency of workers. The difference now is that with a new class of workers, we need new designs. By the year 2000 the work force will be almost as middle-aged as it is young, and we cannot afford to waste the talent of the older worker.

Here are some of the changes Fozard and Popkin see as necessary in designing future work environments:

Lighting: More illumination is required as people grow older, much more than is necessary for younger people. Indeed, a worker of seventy may require almost 100 times as much light as one of twenty to see well when there is glare—as there often is in the modern glass-and-chrome business establishment. Obviously, one solution is to reduce glare. When this is not possible, higher levels of illumination are necessary, and both younger and older workers' efficiency improves with better lighting.

Sudden changes in lighting are more dangerous for older people and may even cause accidents. Most falls occur at the top of a staircase where the lighting is poor. Simply putting a light at the head of stairs can prevent a fall.

Equalized lighting throughout the work area will eliminate sudden dark and light spots, prevent accidents, and increase efficiency. Younger workers will appreciate it too, even though their eyes accommodate to dark and light changes much faster.

Training procedures: This is usually the greatest obstacle to the hiring of older workers. Can they be trained? Will they learn? They can and will—with a little consideration. Consideration of the fact that they might be slower in coming up with answers or might block on familiar names. Much of this difficulty is reduced when anxiety is reduced. For the rest, work training should include memory training.

When it comes to mind-boggling computer counters and read-off tapes, some simplification may be necessary. There are ways of making modern electronics more manageable for older workers by simple adjustments in sequence and structure.

The important thing for management to remember is that by the year 2000, the sixty-year-old worker will be compared with the forty-five-year-old worker rather than the twenty-two-year-old college student in a lab study. Then the older person may not come out so far behind after all, and such changes may be necessary for the majority of the work force.

Motivation: For younger workers this usually means raises, opportunity for advancement, insurance, and other employee benefits. For the older person it usually means only *reassurance that they are capable of doing the work.*

Older workers, and older people in general, attribute any defect in functioning to their "age." They are easily discouraged, and a sense of failure affects even the tasks they are capable of doing as well.

Researchers Fozard and Popkin point out that traditionally industrial psychology has measured abilities, interests, and suitability of personality to a job. They suggest it should be extended to include career changes, prolonging work life, and "planning for a suitable mix of work and leisure during the work span."

This attitude "at the top" would mean that older people will no longer be excluded from normal hiring procedures. They will no longer have to be reassured as to their worth—it will be an established fact. It is already in areas where numbers of older persons have returned to work. It is only in impersonal "big business" and in the modern "corporate world" where the myths persist. But perhaps this will change, too.

After all, a man pushing seventy was recently elected President in the largest landslide of the 20th century, despite all the jokes about his "senility." Age is no obstacle in politics these days, in the United States or elsewhere.

While the job market lags behind in its official concepts and procedures, the federal legislature is raising the retirement age, outlawing "ageism," and taking many other steps (for various reasons, to be sure) which are guaranteed to increase the self-confidence of the older worker.

Bargaining from a Position of Weakness

The older worker is still in this position, of course. Social gerontologist James Dowd, in applying the power-exchange theory to the labor market, points out that older workers not only have less to offer competitively, but what they do have may be devalued simply because of their age. No matter how competent they may be, the burden of proof rests with them because they are older. What older workers do becomes a "test" of what they can do.

The person who has been an expert lathe operator for forty years, must suddenly prove that as retirement age approaches. This situation is not likely to change quickly even in this age of progress for older people. There will probably *not* be a revolt by the older population against this unfair attitude, for there is more than justice involved here.

Profits are not distributed equally. They are distributed proportionately to one's investment; and older people have a great *personal* investment in work, which brings them returns not only in cash, but in self-esteem and increased physical and mental health. So the fact that they may have to "trade down" in the employment world does not affect the profits they still gain from employment.

But there are rumblings. Questions are being raised—not necessarily by today's elderly but tomorrow's. While resentment and opposition may be forestalled in the present generation of elderly, an age-consciousness is developing among the middle-aged which may restore the power balance.

An Age-Segregated Society?

It may seem as if we were heading in that direction, what with the increase of age-segregated communities and the sharpening of issues between young and old. Certainly, from a power-exchange point of view, it may be very good strategy, since age-segregation means equal status, fair exchange, a community of interest, and bargaining from a position of power. In the age-segregated community, an older person is no longer low on the totem pole.

Actually, age-segregation is the pattern for most age groups; children of different ages, adolescents, young adults, middle-aged adults, and the elderly all tend to form distinct social circles. It is only the elderly who are penalized for their age group.

In all age groups, conflicts arise only when there is a crossing over boundaries. So from several points of view, an age-segregated society may be an advantage for the older person. This is not to be confused with institutionalization of the elderly, which is a dehumanizing process imposed on a small segment of the older population who are no longer in a position of choice. The age-segregated community is the exact opposite of institutionalization (although it is sometimes confused with it in the minds of the uninformed), and represents conscious choice on the part of alert, active people who do *not* choose to lose their status or bargaining power in the broader community.

Should age-segregation be stopped? The natural forces of society will determine the outcome. James Dowd views the present trend as resulting from the downgrading of the old, who now find the age-segregated community a place in which to reinstate themselves.

However, Dowd also predicts a future renegotiation between the thirty-five-to-fifty-five-age group and the fifty-five-to-seventy-five-year-olds in which the boundaries between these groups may become nonexistent. The education, health, and continued high-level functioning of the older age group may eventually cause redifinition of the boundary as simply between younger adults and older adults. And there would be no penalty for crossing it.

Young adults are already studying "the adventurous aged," and are interested in the risk-taking lifestyle during the later years. They feel that there is a great deal to be learned about coping skills, functioning, and mental health from the New Elderly.

"Voluntary relocation in later years is no longer seen by them as retiring to 'God's Waiting Room'." Gerontologists are now studying changes in lifestyles, adaptation patterns, and adjustment reactions, not so much for the sake of older adults, but for younger adults who need the information for their own adjustments.

Advantages of Aging

There are many, both for society as a whole and for the New Elderly in particular. Gerontologist Erdman Palmore has listed them. Here are some of those advantages.

First, for society:

Older people are more law abiding. Arrests of people over sixty-five for all offenses comprises only 1.2 percent of total arrests. For felony offenses, it is only 0.5 percent of the total. Not bad for over one-tenth of the population. Except for young children, people over sixty-five are the most law-abiding of all age groups. They represent a reservoir of values and ethics for us all.

They are more involved politically. They vote more frequently, are better informed about public issues, and hold more public offices—including the Presidency.

They do more volunteer work, although surveys show they would prefer paid work. However, for the time being society benefits, since older people do a good job, with or without pay.

They are more vigilant. This may come as a surprise, although it perhaps shouldn't, considering that throughout history older people have traditionally been the watchmen, gatekeepers, and flock-tenders in many societies. Recent studies have shown that older people are more alert to repetitive signals than younger people and are more sensitive to them over a longer period of time. An intruder is less likely to catch them off guard.

Here are some personal advantages for those of us who are aging now:

We are less likely to be victims of crime. We have been led to believe otherwise—elderly victims make good newspaper copy—but the fact is that people over sixty five have much lower victimization rates in nearly all categories of personal crime: robbery, assault, and personal theft. The only crime they suffer from equally is purse-snatching and wallet-stealing.

We have less accidents. The accident rate is less than two-thirds that of all other age groups. It is lower in every category, including motor vehicles, work, and home. The National Safety Council reports that drivers over sixty-five have less accidents and have safer driving records than people under sixty-five. This is only partly due to the fact that they drive less miles per year; the council claims it is also due to more careful driving.

We are in better economic shape. Social Security now covers 90 percent of people over age sixty-five. In addition, government pensions cover all government workers, and private pensions cover almost half of all wage earners in private industry. There is Supplemental Security Income which essentially guarantees a minimum income for everyone over sixty-five and for the handicapped of any age.

Older people pay lower taxes. Property taxes are reduced for people over sixty-five in 80 percent of the states. Double personal exemptions are granted by the federal income tax, and there are many other benefits. It has been estimated that the older population saves about $3.5 billion a year through federal income tax provisions.

There is Medicare. Although it does not cover everything, Medicare and Social Security together are probably the prime reasons for the very existence of the New Elderly today. Not necessarily for what they provide, but for what they imply of the power status of the older person today. There are also free services and reduced rates for various programs, items, and activities too numerous to mention.

Considering the general emphasis on the problems and disadvantages of aging, gerontologist Palmore's optimistic views accentuating the positive come as a welcome change. And one certainly cannot argue with his facts which are statistically based and fully documented.

But is it wise to be optimistic and positive?

The Social Security Backlash
The press reports that younger people are resisting

Social Security taxes and complaining about having to support a nonproductive portion of the population. They are making dangerous sounds, it would seem.

However, when younger people are asked if they prefer to pay taxes or take care of their elderly (and have to be taken care of themselves when they are old), they immediately opt for the taxes. They have no intention of turning the clock back and assuming financial responsibility for their parents or depending on their own children for support when they are old.

Most objections come not from the workers but from the industrial firms whose own contributions increase as the employee's does. Management sees the Social Security tax as a burden on society; the people do not. Actually, the United States is now behind other industrial countries in the portion of the total budget allotted to income maintenance of older people.

Still, it is a dangerous backlash. Fear of aging, and the hostility that always accompanies fear, is still a factor to be reckoned with.

A better solution would be to provide employment for all who want to work and continue income benefits for those who need them.

Aging in the Year 2000

With more people living to be older, by the year 2000 there will be a 50 percent increase in the population over sixty years of age. More important, the *functioning* life span of individuals will continue until shortly before death.

Health, not disease, will be the focus of medical research and services. The goal will be to maintain a person's functioning and prevent disablement and deterioration. When there is a breakdown, advanced rehabilitative medical techniques will restore function to its highest potential.

Loneliness, often viewed as a major problem of aging, will be out of the picture almost entirely. This is happening already, as recent studies show. A survey of several thousand people revealed that the elderly are the *least lonely* of all age groups, even though they are the most likely to live alone.

By the year 2000, the elderly will have more, not less relatives. They will continue to live in separate households, but interdependence, rather than independence, will be the goal. Mutual support systems will replace dependency. Fears of being a "burden" will be replaced by plans for further personality development and expression. There will be plenty of outlets for work and play.

There will be a new kind of woman: one whose identity is based on a self-concept as a worker rather than as a dependent upon a male provider. This will not only ease adjustment to widowhood (which unfortunately will still be a problem in 2000), but will also open up new types of conjoint relationships.

Political participation and power will still be invested in the sixty- to sixty-five year-old group, much as it is in the present. More people will reach their 100-year birthday. Youth will no longer be the criterion in tests of speed and intellectual power.

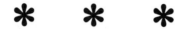

I recently spoke with a seventy-six year-old man who had gone through a series of grueling disappointments and losses. After a period of readjustment he was able to resume his life activities in different form but as rewarding and meaningful as ever.

I told him how much I admired his resilience, his adaptability, his capacity to live life so fully despite misfortune. How did he do it?

"Simple," he said. "Someone, I forget who, once said, *'life is a journey—not necessarily a destination.'* And that's the way I look at it too."

So to him—and all of you—have a wonderful time on your trip.

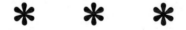

Selected Bibliography

Very long titles are abbreviated.

Chapter One: **You Can Teach an Old Dog New Tricks**

Arenberg, D. "Problem-Solving in Adults." *Journal of Gerontology.* 29 (1974): 650–58.

Birren, J.E., and Schaie, K.W., eds. *Handbook of the Psychology of Aging.* New York: Van Nostrand Reinhold, 1977.

Borger, R., and Seaborne, A. *The Psychology of Learning.* Baltimore: Pelican, 1970.

Botwinick, J., and Storandt, M. "Recall and Recognition in Relation to Age and Sex." *Journal of Gerontology.* 35 (1980): 70–76.

Feier, C.D., and Gerstman, L.J. "Comprehension throughout the Life Span." *Journal of Gerontology.* 35 (1980): 722–28.

Kausler, D.H., and Kleim, D.M. "Age Differences in Processing." *Journal of Gerontology.* 33 (1978): 87–93.

Murrell, F.H. "The Effect of Extensive Practice on Age." *Journal of Gerontology.* 25 (1970): 268–74.

Neugarten, B.L. "Personality and Aging." In Birren, J.E., and Schaie, K.W., eds. *Handbook of the Psychology of Aging.* New York: Van Nostrand Reinhold, 1977.

Powell, R.P. "Psychological Effects of Exercise." *Journal of Gerontology.* 29 (1974): 157–61.

Pribram, K.H. *Brain and Behaviour.* Baltimore: Penguin, 1969.

Pribram, K.H. *On the Biology of Learning.* New York: Harcourt, Brace & World, 1969.

Savage, R.D., et al. *Intellectual Functioning in the Aged.* New York: Barnes & Noble, 1975.

Schwartz, F., and Schiller, P.H. *A Psychoanalytic Model of Attention and Learning.* New York: International Universities Press, 1970.

Woodruff, D.S., and Walsh, D.A. "Research in Adult Learning." *Gerontologist.* 15 (1975): 424–30.

Chapter Two: **The Myth of Senility**

Brody, N. *Personality, Research & Theory.* New York: Academic Press, 1972.

Busse, E.W., and Pfeiffer, E. *Mental Illness in Later Life.* Washington, D.C.: American Psychiatric Association, 1973.

Cohen, G.D. "Research on Aging: A Piece of the Puzzle." *Gerontologist.* 19 (1979): 503–08.

Cohn, V. "Thousands Doomed by False Senility." *Washington Post,* July 17, 1978.

de Rivera, J. *A Structural Theory of the Emotions.* New York: International Universities Press, 1977.

Dudek, S.Z. "Regression in the Service of the Ego." *Journal of Personality Assessment.* 39 (1975): 369–76.

Ernst, P., et. al. "Isolation and the Symptoms of Chronic Brain Syndrome." *Gerontologist.* 18 (1978): 468–74.

Fann, W.E., et al. "Treating the Aged with Psychotropic Drugs." *Gerontologist.* 16 (1976): 322–28.

Folsom, J.C. *Reality Orientation.* American Psychiatric Association, Hospital and Community Psychiatry Service, Washington, D.C., 1975.

Ford, C.V., and Winter, J. "Dementia in Elderly Patients." *Journal of Gerontology.* 36 (1980): 164–69.

Freese, A.S. "Good News About Senility." *Modern Maturity,* February 1978, 9–10.

Jarvik, L.F. "Thoughts on the Psychobiology of Aging." *American Psychologist.* 30 (1975): 576–83.

Katzman, R., et al. *Alzheimer's Disease.* New York: Raven Press, 1978.

McKellar, P. *Mindsplit . . . The Dissociated Self.* London: Dent, 1979.

Pines, M. "Brain Research Sparks Optimism." *APA Monitor,* February, 1981.

———. "Can the Brain Renew Itself?" *Psychology,* American Psychological Association, Washington, D.C., 1977.

Rothschild, D., and Sharp, M.L. "The Origin of Senile Psychosis." *Diseases of the Nervous System.* 2 (1941): 49–54.

Shevrin, H., and Dickman, S. "The Psychological Unconscious." *American Psychologist.* 35 (1980): 421–34.

Tiger, L. *Optimism: The Biology of Hope.* New York: Simon & Schuster, 1979.

Worm-Peterson, J., and Pakkenberg, H. "Atherosclerosis of Cerebral Arteries." *Journal of Gerontology.* 23 (1968): 445–49.

Chapter Three: Memory Loss May Be Good for You

Bartlett, F.C. *Remembering.* Cambridge: Cambridge University Press, 1932.

Botwinick, J., and Storandt, M. *Memory, Related Functions, and Age.* Springfield, Ill.: Charles C. Thomas, 1974.

Bower, G.H. "Mood and Memory." *American Psychologist.* 36 (1981): 129–48.

Brown, M. *Memory Matters.* New York: Crane, Russak, 1977.

Carp, F.M. "On Becoming an Ex-Driver." *Gerontologist.* 7 (1971): 101–3.

Gilbert, J.G., and Levee, R.F. "Patterns of Declining Memory." *Journal of Gerontology.* 26 (1971): 70–75.

Greenwald, A.G. "The Totalitarian Ego." *American Psychologist.* 35 (1980): 603–18.

Jenkins, J.J. "Remember that Old Theory of Memory? Well, Forget It!" *American Psychologist.* 29 (1974): 785–95.

Kail, R.V., and Hagen, J.W. *Perspectives on the Development of Memory.* New Jersey: Erlbaum, 1977.

Kimble, D.P. *The Anatomy of Memory.* Palo Alto: Science and Behavior Books, 1965.

Loftus, E.F., and Loftus, G.R. "On the Permanence of Stored Information in the Human Brain." *American Psychologist.* (1980): 409–20.

Merriam, S. "Function of Reminiscence." *Gerontologist.* 20 (1980): 604–08.

Paul, I.H. *Studies in Remembering.* New York: International Universities Press, 1959.

Pribram, K.H. *Memory Mechanisms.* London: Penguin Books, 1969.

Rapaport, D. *Emotions and Memory.* New York: International Universities Press, 1971.

Reese, H.W. "Life-Span ... Memory," *Gerontologist.* (1973): 472–78.

Schwartz, F., and Rouse, R.O. *The Activation and Recovery of Associations.* New York: International Universities Press, 1961.

Singer, J.L. "Navigating the Stream of Consciousness." *American Psychologist.* 30 (1975): 727–38.

Wallach, H.F., et al. "Memory for Emotional Words." *Journal of Gerontology.* 35 (1980): 371–75.

Chapter Four: Problem Parents of Middle-Aged Children—and Vice Versa

Avant, W.R., and Dressel, P.L. "Perceiving Needs by Staff and Elderly." *Gerontologist.* 20 (1980): 71–77.

Borland, D.C. "Research on Middle-Age." *Gerontologist.* 18 (1978): 379–86.

Estes, C.L. *The Aging Enterprise.* San Francisco: Jossey-Bass, 1979.

Gozali, J. "Age and Attitude." *Gerontologist.* 7 (1971): 289–91.

Halprin, F.B. "Middle-Aged Children and Their Parents." Paper presented at Gerontological Society meeting, Washington, D.C., 1979.

Harris, L., et al. *Myth and Reality of Aging in America.* Washington, D.C.: National Council on Aging, 1975.

Menninger, K. *Whatever Became of Sin?"* New York: Hawthorn, 1975.

Modern Maturity. "More Oldsters Now Disinheriting Children." 1980, Oct/Nov, page 8.

Robinson, B., and Thurnher, M. "Taking Care of Aged Parents." *Gerontologist.* 19 (1979): 586–93.

Shanas, E. "Family Relations of Old People." *Gerontologist.* 19 (1979): 3–9.

Chapter Five: Those Golden Anniversary Blues!

Brandwein, R., et al. "The Married Widow(er)." Paper presented at Gerontological Society meeting, Washington, D.C., 1979.

Danis, B., and Noelker, L. "The World of Never-Married Older Women." Paper presented at Gerontological Society meeting, Washington, D.C., 1979.

Dickinson, M.W. "Mid-Life Divorce: Invitation to Trauma." *Los Angeles Times,* April 17, 1980.

Dowd, J.J. "Aging as Exchange." *Journal of Gerontology.* 30 (1975): 584–94.

Glick, P.C. "Future Marital Status and Living Arrangements of the Elderly." *Gerontologist.* 3 (1979): 124–30.

Havighurst, R.J. "Adapting to Old Age." *Gerontologist.* 8, (1968): 67–71.

Smith, D. "Long-Married Pairs Share Unhappiness." *Los Angeles Times.* June 22, 1980.

Time. "Not So Merry Widowers." August 10, 1981, p. 45.

Troll, L.E. "Approval of Spouse in Middle Age." *Proceedings, 77th Annual Convention.* American Psychological Association, 1969.

Chapter Six: Dealing With Depression in Everyday Life

Beck, A.T. *Depression.* New York: Harper & Row, 1967.

Durlak, J.A. "Attitudes Toward Life and Death." *Journal of Consulting and Clinical Psychology.* 38 (1972): 463–70.

Farberow, N.L., and Moriwaki, S.Y. "Self-Destructive Crises in the Older Person." *Gerontologist,* August 1975, 333–37.

Frankl, V.E. *The Doctor and the Soul.* New York: Knopf, 1965.

Huesmann, L.R. "Learned Helplessness as a Model of Depression." *Journal of Abnormal Psychology.* 87 (special issue), 1978.

Jarvik, L.F., and Russell, D. "Anxiety, Aging and the Third Emergency Reaction." *Journal of Gerontology.* 34 (1979): 197–200.

Lewinsohn, P.M., et al. *Control Your Depression.* New Jersey: Prentice-Hall, 1978.

Miller, M. "Geriatric Suicide." *Gerontologist.* 18, (1978): 488–95.

Preston, C.E., and Williams, R.H. "Views of the Aged on the Timing of Death." *Gerontologist.* Winter, 1971.

Salter, C.A., and Salter, C. "Attitudes Toward Aging and Death Anxiety." *Gerontologist.* 16 (1976): 232–36.

Seligman, M.E.P. *Helplessness: On Depression, Development, and Death.* San Francisco: Freeman, 1975.

Templer, D.I. "Death Anxiety, Depression and Health of Retired Persons." *Journal of Gerontology.* 26 (1971): 521–23.

Timnick, L. "Scientists Hope to Lift Elderly Spirits." *Los Angeles Times,* March 13, 1980.

Chapter Seven: Food, Friends, Exercise— The Big Three of Aging

Arthritis Foundation. "Understanding the 'Fibrositis' Syndrome." *Bulletin on the Rheumatic Diseases.* 28 (1977–78 series). Atlanta.

Beller, S., and Palmore, E. "Longevity in Turkey, *Gerontologist, Spring.* (1974): 373–76.

Elsayed, M., et al. "Cognitive Functioning and Exercise." *Journal of Gerontology.* 35 (1980): 383–87.

Freeman, J.T. "Posture in the Aging and Aged Body." *Journal of the American Medical Association.* 165 (1957): 843–46.

———. "Stress and Senescence." *Journal of the American Geriatrics Society.* 7 (1959).

———. "Of Aging and Illness." *Journal of Geriatric Psychiatry.* 1 (1968): 263–73.

Jarvik, L.F. "Thoughts on the Psychobiology of Aging." *American Psychologist.* 30 (1975): 576–83.

Jewett, S.P. "The Longevity Syndrome." *Gerontologist.* (1973): 91–99.

Kyuicharyants, V. "Will the Human Life-Span Reach 100?" *Gerontologist.* (1974): 377–80.

Medvedev, Z.A. "Longevity: A Biological or Social Problem?" *Gerontologist.* (1974): 381–87.

Palmore, E.B., and Stone, V. "Predictors of Longevity." *Gerontologist.* 1973: 88–90.

Sherwood, S. "Senility, a Mask for Nutritional Deficiencies." *Geriatric Focus.* April, 1973: 3–4.

Spirduso, W.W. "Physical Fitness: Aging and Speed." *Journal of Gerontology.* 35 (1980): 850–65.

Ward, R.A. "The Never-Married in Later Life." *Journal of Gerontology.* 34 (1979): 861–69.

Chapter Eight: Swinging after Sixty

Busse, E.W. "Sexual Attitudes and Behavior in the Elderly." *Geriatric Focus.* 12 (1972).

Dean, S.T. "Those 'Dirty Old Men—Just Sexy Senior Citizens." *Geriatric Focus.* 12 (1973).

Francher, J.S., and Henkin, J. "The Menopausal Queen." *American Journal of Orthopsychiatry.* 43. (1973): 670–74.

Freeman, J.T. "Sexual Aspects of Aging." In Cowdry, E.V., ed., *Care of the Geriatric Patient.* St. Louis: Mosby, 1971.

Karacan, I., et al. "Nocturnal Penile Tumescence in Elderly Males." *Journal of Gerontology.* 27 (1972): 39–45.

Laner, M.R. "Growing Older Male: Heterosexual and Homosexual." *Gerontologist.* 18 (1978): 496–99.

Loughman, C. "Eros and the Elderly." *Gerontologist.* 20 (1980): 182–87.

Ludeman, K. "The Sexuality of the Older Person." *Gerontologist.* 21 (1981): 203–08.

Masters, W.H., and Johnson, V.E. *Human Sexual Response.* Boston: Little Brown, 1966.

———. *Human Sexual Inadequacy.* Boston: Little Brown, 1970.

Miller, M.B., et al. "Family and Sexual Conflict." *Gerontologist.* August 1975: 291–96.

Odegard, W., and Deskin, K. "Sexual Growth in Aging and Illness." Virginia: Veterans Administration Publications, 1977.

Plutchik, R., et al. "Studies of Body Image." *Journal of Gerontology.* 33 (1978): 68–75.

Rossman, I. "Sexual Function During Advanced Age." In Finkel, L.P., ed. *Clinical Geriatrics.* Philadelphia: Lippencott, 1971.

Treas, J., and Van Hilst, A. "Marriage and Remarriage Among Older Americans, *Gerontologist.* 16 (1976): 132–36.

Chapter Nine: What Kind of Old Person Will You Be?

Bloom, M., et al. "Interviewing the Aged." *Gerontologist.* Winter, 1971.

Bultena, G.L., and Powers, E.A. "Denial of Aging." *Journal of Gerontology.* 33 (1978): 748-54.

Longino, C.F., et al. "The Aged Subculture." *Journal of Gerontology.* 35 (1980): 758-67.

Machover, Karen. *Personality Projection in the Drawing of the Human Figure.* Springfield, Ill.: Charles C. Thomas, 1949.

Oberleder, M. "An Attitude Scale to Determine Adjustment in ... the Aged." *Journal of Chronic Disease.* 15 (1962): 915-23.

Palmore, E., et al. "Stress and Adaptation in Later Life." *Journal of Gerontology.* 34 (1979): 841-51.

Walsh, R.P., and Connor, C.L. "Old Men and Young Women." *Journal of Gerontology.* 34 (1979): 561-68.

Chapter Ten: Meet the New Elderly

Abercrombie, R.K. "A Right to Die." *Gerontologist.* 21 (1981): 17.

Brickner, P.W., et al. "Home Maintenance for the Home-Bound Aged." *Gerontologist.* 16 (1976): 25-29.

Dowd, J.J. "Exchange Rates and Old People." *Journal of Gerontology.* 35 (1980): 596-602.

Engel, J.B., and Charles, D.C. "Aging and Alienation: A Fresh Look." Paper presented at Gerontological Society meeting, Washington, D.C., 1979.

Fozard, J.L., and Popkin, S.J. "Optimizing Adult Development." *American Psychologist.* November, 1978.

Greene, B. "The Elderly Beached by Life's Ebbing Tide." *Los Angeles Times,* April 6, 1980.

Harris L., et. al. *Myth and Reality of Aging in America.* National Council on Aging, Washington, D.C., 1975.

Hellebrandt, F.A. "A New Look at the Sterotypes of the Elderly." *Gerontologist.* 20 (1980): 404–17.

Horowitz, J. "Recycling Grandparents as Parents." Los Angeles Times, May 4, 1980.

Kalish, R.A. "Grandparents and Divorce." Paper presented at the Gerontological Society meeting, Washington, D.C., 1979.

Neugarten, B. "Acting One's Age: New Rules For Old." *Psychology Today.* April, 1980: 66–80.

Neugarten, B.L. "The Future and the Young-Old." *Gerontologist.* 15 (1975): 4–9.

Palmore, E. "Advantages of Aging." *Gerontologist.* 19 (1979): 220–23.

Revenson, T.A., and Rubenstein, C. "Debunking the Myth of Loneliness in Old Age." Paper presented at Gerontological Society meeting, San Diego, 1980.

Stephen, B. "Aging Parents: Handwriting on the Wall." *Los Angeles Times,* November 9, 1980.

Uhlenberg, P. "Changing Structure of the Older Population of the USA During the 20th Century." *Gerontologist.* 17 (1977): 197–203.

Index

Divorce 44, 69, 87, 89, 98, 100, 157, 159
Dowd, James, J. 92-3, 102, 191, 193
Down Syndrome 36

Education 19, 28, 32, 33, 55, 180, 182, 183
Emerson, R.W. 35
Entrapment 170
Estes, Carroll L. (*The Aging Enterprise*) 73

Ferenczi, Sandor 15
Fozard, James L. 188-91
Frankl, V.E. 126
Freeman, J.T. 133, 141
Freud, Sigmund 14, 15, 106, 156
Franklin, Benjamin 105

Goethe, J.W. 163
Grandparents 76, 79, 81, 184, 185-6
Gray Panthers 76
Great Depression 86

Harris Poll 179, 183
Healing Brain 32 (renews itself) 40
Hemlock Society 120-1
Homosexuality 150, 159-60
Hormones 33, 56, 125

Identification 78, 82, 96, 97

Jarvik, Lissy 144
Jung, Carl 14, 15

Kinsey, A. 147

LaLanne, Jack 20
Libido 34, 112, 156
Living Will 84
Longitudinal studies 28, 31
Low calorie diet 128-130

Marital singlehood 101
Masturbation 147
Media (effect of) 69, 71, 72
Medicare 195
Menninger, Karl 72
Memory control 58-9
Miami Beach 71, 79, 181
Moses, Grandma 20

Narcissistic supplies 107-8
Neugarten, Bernice 20, 184-5

Oberleder Attitude Scale 163
Oxygen therapy 37

Palmore, Erdman 193
Popkin, S.J. 188-91
Power (loss of) 80-2, 83-4, 86-8, 100
Power (exchange theory) 92-4, 191
Power (group) 171-2

210   Index

Suggested Reading

The Retirement Money Book
New Ways You Can Have More Income
DESPITE INFLATION

• Real Estate • Securities • Insurance •
Barter • New Careers

by Ferd Nauheim

Whether you are planning for retirement, or already
there, it is practically impossible to read this clear and
practical book without discovering a variety of ways to
have more income throughout your retirement years.
• Where to look for investment growth potential

• How judicious spending in retirement is more important
  than saving

• The seven answers to "I have no capital."

• How to give yourself cost-of-living increases

• How to take advantage of the increased value of your
  home

"It s coverage and clarity are great."

—Arthur F. Bouton, President-Elect American Association of Retired Persons

ISBN 87491-437-X/$11.95 hardcover
250 pages, 6 x 9, index

ACROPOLIS BOOKS LTD.,   2400 17th St. N.W.,   Washington, D.C. 2000

Cut Your Grocery Bills in Half!

Supermarket Survival

by Barbara Salsbury with Cheri Loveless

Americans spend twice what they should on food, according to these two savvy consumer advocates. In **CUT YOUR GROCERY BILLS IN HALF** they challenge some of our most time-honored ways to save money—like coupons and refunding. They offer new, practical ways to cope with the ever soaring cost of food and commodities, inside the supermarket and at home.

CUT YOUR GROCERY BILLS delves into what manufacturers, advertisers, brokers, grocers and computerized cash registers do to your food costs. The authors teach you how to use your knowledge of marketing techniques to "take advantage" of the supermarket, for a change.

You'll learn all the trade secrets of these smart shoppers from buying in bulk to deciding where to shop, to how to read ads, to in-store psychology. Learn how to buy the product, not the package; how to choose a brand, plan meals around the seasons, form a co-op, even make some of your own groceries.

Each chapter includes personal workbook pages for storing your own important money-saving tips and discoveries. The authors' practical shopping tips are featured in easy-to-read lists, divided by food groups and non-food groups.

CUT YOUR GROCERY BILLS IN HALF! is guaranteed to do just that. It's your guide to supermarket survival. Try it in your household.

> **Without coupons, gimmicks, or sacrifices, I have spent less than half what other families of four pay for groceries. I've done it for ten years and even bought the brands I like. I guarantee that you can do it, too.**
>
> *Barbara Salsbury*

Barbara Salsbury and Cheri Loveless

Barbara Salsbury is the author of four previous books and numerous articles. She lectures extensively on supermarket survival. Mrs. Salsbury became interested in this topic when she was forced to feed her own family of four on $5,000 a year. She did it.

Cheri Loveless is a homemaker and writer. She is the author of several articles and the *Northern Virginia Consumers' Co-op Handbook*. Mrs. Loveless is the mother of four children, and daughter of columnist, Jack Anderson.

ISBN 87491-531-7/$7.95 quality paper
200 pages, 8 x 9, illustrated, index

CROPOLIS BOOKS LTD.,   2400 17th St. N.W.,   Washington, D.C. 20009

Health After 40

Mental and Physical Fitness
in the Prime of Your Life

by Robert Taylor, M.D.

Previously published as "Welcome to the Middle Years,"
HEALTH AFTER 40 offers sensible solutions to many
common problems of the prime years, and helps point the
way to meeting the challenges of middle age. Says
Publishers Weekly, "Here's a sensible, compassionate
physician whose advice can make a real difference in the
reader's life . . . He [Taylor] confronts the facts and
fallacies of the aging process and offers reasonable
suggestions for making the mid-years the prime of life."

Dr. Robert Taylor is Associate Professor, Department of
Family and Community Medicine, Bowman Gray School
of Medicine, Wake Forest University.

ISBN 87491-530-9/$6.95 quality paper
206 pages, 6 × 9, bibliography, index

Win the Happiness Game

by Dr. William G. Nickels

foreword by Dr. Warren Johnson

"I am impressed by *WIN THE HAPPINESS GAME.* It
offers sound and workable suggestions for finding real
fulfillment in life. Since it made me happy just to read the
book, one would surely develop deeper joy following Dr.
Nickels' wise thoughts."   **—Dr. Norman Vincent Peale**

Dr. Nickels, a long time student of self-help techniques,
offers a systematic approach to . . .

- Schedule time for more things you like to do
- Discover joy in everyday occurrences and live for
  "now"
- Get more out of vacations and free time
- Solve problems, be more assertive, get in touch with
  your feelings

Happiness is a skill you can learn—and share with others!

ISBN 87491-070-6/$11.95 hardcover
ISBN 87491-528-8/$6.95 quality paper
200 pages, 6 x 9, index

ACROPOLIS BOOKS LTD.,   2400 17th St. N.W.,   Washington, D.C. 200

The New 15 Minute Gourmet

150 Recipes You Can Prepare in 15 Minutes . . .
or Less PLUS 108 Quick Tips for Giving
any Meal an Elegant Flair

by Beverly Ann Adams

Back by popular demand, this handy little cookbook is
guaranteed to free any cook from the kitchen. In less than
15 minutes—each of the 150 delicious new recipes can be
easily prepared.

This revised edition of the ever popular *15 Minute
Gourmet* contains new recipes for hors d'oeuvres, soups,
main dishes, breads, vegetables, desserts, drinks plus 108
quick and different tips to make every meal an elegant,
festive occasion.

The entertaining tips alone are worth the price of **THE
NEW 15 MINUTE GOURMET**, and there are also tips
for dieters, microwave recipes, fanciful toasts and drink
recipes.

ISBN 87491-490-6/$4.95 quality paper
120 pages, 6 x 9, illustrated

The Stress FoodBook

The Natural Way to Fight Stress

by Margaret C. Dean, M.S., R.D.
illustrated by Loel Barr

Today everyone lives under stress. It is a constant
factor in our lives, and some stress is good for you. It
motivates you to act. But when there is too much stress,
or it lasts too long, it affects your health.

But now there is **THE STRESS FOODBOOK** in which
noted nutritionist Margaret Dean tells you how to manage
stress through diet. She offers two complete diets: "The
Stress Relief Diet" and "The Stress Prevention Diet". Now
you can begin to relieve your tension by strengthening
your body.

Use **THE STRESS FOODBOOK** as your personal
program for managing stress. Feeling good, you'll be able
to use the challenges of stressful situations to your
advantage, instead of being overwhelmed by them.

ISBN 87491-089-7/$12.95 hardcover
ISBN 87491-295-4/$6.95 quality paper
128 pages, 8 x 9, illustrations

ACROPOLIS BOOKS LTD.,   2400 17th St. N.W.,   Washington, D.C. 20009

Stretch!

The Lazy Person's Exercise Book
The Active Person's Relaxation Book

by Ann Smith

Children and animals stretch instinctively to maintain
their muscle tone and circulation—but most adult exercise
programs concentrate only on achieving muscle strength
. . . not the elasticity we need.

Now in **STRETCH!, Ann Smith,** an experienced dance
and physical education teacher, has created a system of
stretch exercises that prepare adults for any physical or
recreational sport by developing their flexibility.

Whatever your age or condition, this total fitness
program will free your mind and body from the blahs
and get you in shape for swimming, jogging, tennis,
dance—you name it!

ISBN 87491-239-3/$6.95 quality paper
176 pages, 8 x 9, fully illustrated

Choices of a Growing Woman

by Maggie S. Davis

CHOICES OF A GROWING WOMAN is a woman-to-
woman book about choices. The book is a testimony to
the author's belief that no matter how much money a
woman makes, no matter what her age or state of mind,
she can always choose to start moving in directions that
feel better to her.

Each chapter is not a chapter—but an exploration of a
specific choice . . .

Choice #1: To Believe in My Own Power

Choice #2: To Treat Myself Royally

Choice #3: To Reach Out to Others

Choice #4: To Stop Sabotaging My Decisions

Choice #5: To Take Risks

Choice #6: To Forget My Age

Maggie S. Davis

Maggie Davis, a doctor's daughter, has been a mediator,
counselor, trainer, teacher, waitress, poet, editor, writer.

ISBN 87491-418-3/$7.95 hardcover title "Blooming"
ISBN 87491-525-2/$4.95 quality paper
132 pages, 5-1/2 x 8-1/2 illustrated

ACROPOLIS BOOKS LTD.,   2400 17th St. N.W..   Washington, D.C. 20009